P9-EDL-895

Menopause

A GUIDE FOR WOMEN
AND THE MEN WHO LOVE THEM

MENOPAUSE

A Guide for Women
and the Men Who Love Them

Winnifred Berg Cutler, Ph.D.
Celso-Ramón García, M.D.
David A. Edwards, Ph.D.

W · W · NORTON & COMPANY, New York · London

Published simultaneously in Canada by George J. McLeod Limited, Toronto.
Printed in the United States of America.

The text of this book is composed in 11/13 Avanta, with display type set in Bauer Bodoni.
Composition and manufacturing by The Hadden Craftsmen, Inc.
Book design by A. Christopher Simon

First Edition

LIBRARY OF CONGRESS CATALOGING IN PUBLICATION DATA

Cutler, Winnifred Berg.
  Menopause, a guide for women and the men who
love them.
  Includes index.
  1. Menopause.   I. García, Celso-Ramón, 1921–
II. Edwards, David A.   III. Title.
RG186.C93 1983   618.1'75   82–18975

ISBN 0-393-01709-5

W. W. Norton & Company, Inc., 500 Fifth Avenue, New York, N.Y. 10110
W. W. Norton & Company Ltd., 37 Great Russell Street, London WC1B 3NU

1 2 3 4 5 6 7 8 9 0

Contents

Illustrations

Illustrations by CAROLINE MEINSTEIN

11

12 *ILLUSTRATIONS*

Preface

For women living into their mid-forties, the menopause is a fact of life. The decision to write a book about the menopause grew out of our conviction that knowledge has recently expanded in the areas of aging and hormones and that women wanted to know, frankly and fully, the state of this knowledge.

One of us (Dr. Cutler) is a reproductive biologist who is actively engaged in research about healthy menopausal women. She is also a mother of teenage children. Another (Dr. García) is a practicing gynecological reproductive endocrinologist and surgeon who serves as the medical director of the Division of Human Reproduction at the Hospital of the University of Pennsylvania. He was also the 1982 president of the American Fertility Society, a gynecological research and teaching forum. He is a husband and father whose clinical and personal experiences include the menopausal years. Dr. Edwards is a professor of psychology at Emory University, where he teaches classes in psychobiology and human sexuality and conducts research dealing with the relationship between hormones and behavior.

This book spans many disciplines, including medicine, reproductive physiology, endocrinology, metabolism, biochemistry, epidemiology, sociology, anthropology, and psychology. There is a large professional literature that covers various aspects of menopause. This book has its roots in that literature, and throughout the text we cite many of the references upon which we have drawn in forming our conclusions. Of necessity we have used some terms that are probably unfamiliar to most readers and have, therefore, provided a glossary at the end of the book in which these terms are defined.

In the fall of 1979, after having secured funds from the National Institute of Health, the Stanford Menopause Project was established at Stanford University jointly by Dr. Julian Davidson, a distinguished neuroendocrinologist, and Dr. Winnifred Cutler. The study was the first of its kind in the United States and was designed to evaluate normal, healthy women as they passed through the menopause. In order to recruit subjects, Dr. Cutler appeared briefly on radio and television talk shows and explained that a study of menopause was getting under way. She described to the broadcast listeners the need for healthy women who were approaching their menopause and asked them to get involved in the project so that the process of menopause could be carefully studied.

Dr. Cutler asked for the volunteers to serve either as data collectors or as participants. It was requested that they call her office at Stanford. The response was great. For two weeks the phones rang continuously with offers of help. Several hundred women were enrolled, twenty of them as research assistants, the rest as research subjects. Although Dr. Cutler has returned to her work in Pennsylvania, today, the project still continues under the direction of Dr. Norma McCoy and Dr. Julian Davidson. Some of the original participants involved in the project continue to be studied as they advance deeper into their menopause.

A great many of the research subjects described the details of their personal searches to understand what was happening to them as they approached menopause. They felt frustrated as they sought, but were unable to find, books from libraries and bookstores that would provide accurate and understandable information on menopause. Many of them joined the study in hopes of finding answers to their questions, answers that were not in books. Many also described their despair and frustration at the treatment (or lack of treatment) offered by their doctors when they sought help (or information) about their hot flashes, loss of a sense of well-being, sagging skin, or vaginal distress during coitus. Because of these frustrating experiences, many of the women who participated in the project asked Dr. Cutler to write a book for people like themselves. They wanted a reference to help answer the questions they were asking. This book was written not only for those women but for all women who may share the desire to learn about themselves. It was also written for the husbands, sons, and brothers, who as part of the family will find such information important in living with the women they love.

We bring to the book a sense of mission: to offer to our readers the detailed information they will need to understand menopause and maximize health care. Here men will also find important information about their own changes in sexuality as well as the information that will help them comprehend the uniquely feminine experience of menopause.

We hope that you will find this book helpful. If you find it too simple or too complicated, please understand that each reader brings a different educational background to the reading. We tried to write it for readers who have an inquiring mind but no scientific background. After you finish the book, you may discover that some of your questions remain unanswered. There is still a great deal to be learned about the menopause, and we encourage you to share your questions as well as your reactions to the book. Please write to us c/o Dr. Winnifred Cutler, Box 214, Haverford,

Pennsylvania 19104. We would like to hear from you, and although we may be unable to personally answer all mail, we *will* use your comments to guide us in planning future research.

WINNIFRED BERG CUTLER
CELSO-RAMÓN GARCÍA
DAVID A. EDWARDS

Preface for Men

If you are like most men, the term "menopause" probably has little objective meaning for you beyond the fact that you know it marks the end of a woman's reproductive years. You may even think that this is a specifically female subject and have avoided becoming informed about it. Even so, if you are living with a woman going through her menopausal transition, the chances are good that you will have had some firsthand exposure to menopausal symptoms before much time has passed. Although some people use the term "male menopause" to describe parallel changes that men undergo, such a term is misleading. Male and female reproductive physiology are critically different. While men produce a fresh supply of sperm each day, often into advanced age, women are *born* with *all* the eggs they will ever have. These eggs get used up through time. Menopause describes the end (pause) of the egg-releasing menstrual years. Other details of male gonadal changes are described in Chapter 7; the changes in a woman's gonadal physiology are described in Chapters 1 and 2.

Does the woman in your life start sweating suddenly without apparent cause? Drenched with sweat, she may wake you up in the night, needing to change the linen to get dry again. Sexually she may not seem responsive to you. She may seem to have lost her interest in sex, and when you do have intercourse—she may have pain. If so, what you are seeing are symptoms commonly experienced by women going through the change of life. And there are other symptoms, too, described in Chapter 3. If your partner's symptoms are distressing to you, imagine what they must be like for her.

Menopausal distress can affect the quality of a relationship between a man and a woman. *How informed you are does make a difference.* Consider this scenario. A woman is distressed because she is experiencing profound physical and emotional discomforts (hot flashes, night sweats, sexual discomfort, etc.). She complains. Her partner is upset because he doesn't understand what is happening. The stable routine of a middle-aged couple can be shattered. The more upset he becomes, the more defensive she becomes. He accuses. She reacts. She feels doubly oppressed —first by the profound physical experience she is going through, and second by the sinking sense of betrayal by her unaware and unhelpful man. Even a good relationship can be stressed by such a sequence. Here is what one fifty-four-year-old woman had to say after thirty-seven years of marriage:

I tire easily; hot flashes night and day; sweating and headaches. . . . Sexual activity occurs once a week if I really make myself for my husband's sake though we had a great sex life before and I was always very receptive. . . . Maybe this has no bearing on anything, but I must admit my husband was extremely unsympathetic about my whole problem. The last two or three months he has tried to understand my feelings. He felt the hot flashes and feelings that went with them were pure figments of my imagination. Because I suppose he knew how loving I had always been in the past, but he just couldn't or wouldn't understand. He was certain that I was "holding back." . . . My doctor finally decided I should try these pills for a couple of months to see if some of my discomfort would leave. I do find that the flushes are less. . . . I had hoped to find out why or if it is possible for this menopause to mess up, what was before, a lovely life—it is very distressing to me and it infuriates my husband.

Although a woman's menopausal difficulties can seem to come from nowhere, they are *not* imaginary. They are real. They herald the menopausal transition. And she may not even know what is happening or that these upsets are as natural and as predictable for the vast majority of women as the changing of the seasons are in nature. She may not appreciate how others perceive her. She may look normal but behave strangely because of how she feels. As you become informed, you will be alert to her distress and can help her overcome difficulties. At least she will have you on her side.

As a woman passes through her forties, her physiology changes. These are described in Chapters 1 and 2. In large part the symptoms of the change of life are the result, and these are described in Chapter 3. Although menopausal symptoms are a natural part of the aging process for the vast majority of women, you should not assume that you and she are helpless. In fact, appropriate medical treatment can alleviate or prevent those menopausal symptoms that have their roots in a woman's changing physiology.

You do have some control. With knowledge, you can materially affect the process, shorten it, and turn it around from distress to comfort. If you understand what is happening, your help can be critically important. Your emotional support has the power to provide a climate for correcting some of the difficulties of this period. Your love, concern, and informed help can mean a lot. With awareness, you can help her seek out effective medical aid.

Your efforts during this time of stress can help your relationship to grow. You can turn this major life experience into a marvelous opportunity to understand her and to enrich her appreciation of you. The woman who is blessed with an understanding and emotionally supportive partner—one who takes the trouble to become informed—is likely to give back far more than she was given.

This book is designed to help women and men to become informed about the menopause. In it you will find chapters that explain what the change of life is and how hormone changes during this period produce a cluster of distressing symptoms. You will find a chapter about bones and osteoporosis, a very serious bone disease that develops in about 50 percent of women over the age of sixty. Osteoporosis is related to the hormone changes of menopause. You will find out how hormone treatment alleviates menopausal symptoms and prevents the development of osteoporosis, and you will find information about the risks of hormone treatment and how these risks can be reversed. The woman in your life may one day have to face making a decision about having a hysterectomy. You will find a chapter which describes the surgery and some of the problems which can result from it.

Taking responsibility for one's health is critically important to a well-lived and happy existence. Both the man and the woman need to maintain their health and to be supportive of each other in order to enjoy the fruits of their life after fifty.

In this book you will find the facts you may need about the menopause. They have been drawn from our intense study of the scientific and biomedical literature. Throughout the book you will find two related perspectives presented: the facts from the biomedical studies and *the actual words of women* who have experienced these situations and are describing how they felt at the time. If you listen to both, you can better understand the menopausal experience.

The uniquely feminine phenomenon of the menopause affects both women and the men who love them.

Menopause

A GUIDE FOR WOMEN
AND THE MEN WHO LOVE THEM

Introduction

The ways in which women experience menopause are as varied as women themselves. For some it is a gentle variation in the rhythms of their lives, its effects minimal. For others, its effects are pronounced, sometimes difficult, but they can be coped with. For still others, however, "the change" has devastating physical and emotional consequences.

Most women experience menopause "naturally," the first signs usually appearing when the women are in their early forties (although the signs may appear even sooner). For others, though, menopause comes abruptly and prematurely when, in their thirties or even twenties, they undergo hysterectomies.

Throughout this book we will be alternating between the actual voices of menopausal women and those of the authors. First, some women speak.

The onset of irregular periods came in this last year, and the periods I do have are heavy, with some clotting and discom-

fort. I tend to also have a few days of the "blues," feeling
of frustration and some fatigue. My libido has always been
healthy, and the only physical symptom that I have noticed
is that my hair is starting to turn grey and I must watch my
diet more carefully, as the midline seems to take on weight.
I consider menstrual cycles a normal part of my life, and I
have always been and still am physically very active. I feel
exercise is extremely important for me in keeping my whole
personality in balance. I swim, hike, ski, skate, play racket-
ball with or without a period. I have noticed some change
in my general attitude to life—but I am not sure that it is
due to the "change." My life has been so full of "changes"
in the last five years that I find it hard to pinpoint one that
has more importance than another. The painful divorce, the
loss of income, finding my way as a single person at 50,
surviving financially in an inflationary market, managing the
entire routine of business, home, and property, social life,
sex life, and concern about how to stay healthy are challenging and are all possible sources for the feelings of the blahs.
I am gregarious with many friends—young and old—and I
do not see behavioral changes in myself, except that my
sense of humor has increased and I am more critical of
events and people who waste my time or spirit.

[I had an] overwhelming feeling of being stifled and suffo-
cating night sweats; couldn't stand to touch my breasts due
to tenderness and heaviness; insomnia which remains a
problem; leg aches in the night particularly; backache; overwhelming feelings of anxiety which made me feel sick to my
stomach; headaches often intense and often accompanied
by worse nausea. . . . My life became intolerable and I felt
(feel) I had to save myself. [I] have good relationships with
friends and co-workers. Adjusting has been (and is, though
less) very difficult—and get[s me] very depressed—but con-

sciously keep very busy with work and taking classes and get completely exhausted.

My husband implies he really "never got enough" from me but I don't believe this is true as my remembrances include much tenderness and sexual enjoyment. I do not have much sexual desire right now but I do miss touching and closeness at night.

I am now 62 years old and in fairly good health. My experience with the menopause lasted about 10–12 years. My gynecologist refused to give me any medication during this period. It was a time of uncomfortableness for me, especially through the winters. At several periods from October through January I had "hot flashes" every half hour, day and night. The perspiration ran down my temples and back. ... My office mates couldn't believe what they saw. But after having what was happening explained thoroughly to me by my doctor I accepted his decision. I feel many times medication is possibly harmful and readily available to women who are so spoiled by conveniences that they just do not want to be annoyed by "Nature's" body changes. The biggest drawback is the sad situation between mothers and daughters who do not "talk" about our body processes at an early age —knowing something as "natural" as a child can form attitudes that last us through our lives and help us through trying times.

About a year ago hot flashes began and grew very severe. Sleep was interrupted continually. Clothes absolutely soaked through. Kept changes of night clothes by bedside. In August, September and October flashes were almost regularly [coming] every 40 minutes. ... Knew when the onslaught was approaching and nothing could be done to stop it. Absolutely felt like I would burn up. Beads of moisture *would pour out of pores on breast area, around waistline, back of neck, forehead, above lip line. You could actually see droplets standing and running. Anyone touching body would receive reaction that "I was on fire." Flash would last approximately 3 to 5 minutes and moisture would disappear! Did not have odor. Usual places like underarms were completely free of this flash. . . . Most embarrassing to be in a business conference eyeball to eyeball with executive and suffer through a flash and try to respond normally as if nothing had happened.*

After a highly satisfying sexual life with same partner (husband) it has been rather upsetting and distressing to find my libido is subsiding. My husband is having trouble in holding an erection which he is most concerned about. He has the desire but cannot respond. Also in the past year, hot flashes have been occurring during intercourse—most distressing to both partners. Have been so absorbed in climbing business ladder successfully, I do not have desire for sex as much and this could be because of my husband's problem and concern over his possible feeling of depression and hurt at not being able to perform as usual. We are a very close couple.

My premature change occurred at the age of 42 due to a hysterectomy and I have been taking estrogen ever since. I'm now 60 years of age and still taking estrogen which helps relieve the hot flashes. I still have those occasional sweating periods but not for long periods of time and not too unbearable. Other than these flashes, the changes one talks about aren't such an obvious thing. Certain changes in the pigmentation occur, causing brown spots on the skin. As far as sexual activity, there are not changes as it is the same as always. Certainly as one gets older, there may be less frequency, but no less qualitatively.

*I became a widow at the age of 43 just when I began
menopause. . . . I have been celibate since my husband's
death. I cannot say with certainty my state of mind is due
to my body's changes or the many adjustments I have made
these past few years. However, for what it's worth, here it
is: I often feel cheated because I am a widow. I was looking
forward to menopause—then I could relax and enjoy having
a relationship with my husband. Until that time I was always
a little uneasy about having sex because of the worry of
pregnancy (I used only suppositories and/or prophylactics).
Having two beautiful children, I did not want any more. I
find that I still have a sex drive. Although it has no direct
outlet, I channel my energies into other things. I have always
had a good rapport with men and I continue to have male
friends with whom I go out occasionally. I don't think menopause should interfere with or affect one's sex life. If anything, it should enhance it because one is more experienced,
with fewer inhibitions or fears. . . . I must confess that my
patience has shortened considerably, especially toward older
people, for whom I had endless patience. I wonder if this
due to the fact that I am now older.*

Before the change superficial conversation was adequate
with friends. I liked just skimming over topics at bridge
table. Impressing them with desserts I made seemed important or how my home looked or giving that Christmas party,
etc. Now bridge-group–type entertainment and conversation is intolerable. Take me as I am is more my style now.
I'm more comfortable with myself and no longer need to
impress others. Don't like to entertain any more—prefer to
just be home or on a drive with my husband. Before, I just
wanted to get involved in everything, couldn't seem to say
no. Ego played a big part in what I did. Now I can say No!

Want to commit myself to less (committee chairmanships etc.). Need time to just let me enjoy and relax more, doing things I like without pressure.

I was two years past my last period and feeling so badly that I had to take a leave from my job. At that point I was desperate for any information on the subject [of menopause]. I was extremely tired most of the time and feeling very nervous. I was experiencing hot flashes six or seven times at night, which interrupted my sleep, and several times each day. In a three-year period, I had been to two family practitioners (one of whom was my family doctor) and two gynecologists. The first three gave me complete physicals which cost upwards of $100 each, and two referred me to a psychiatrist. I saw the psychiatrist three times for a cost of $155, even though I was convinced that my problem was physical. The third gynecologist, a heavy-set woman with mustache, told me to "tough it out." I later learned from another doctor that she frequently told young people that the only way to prevent pregnancy was to refrain from intercourse. The second physician suggested a course in assertiveness training. I cried a lot after the operation [a hysterectomy performed at the age of 38; she is now 51] or when I got home from the hospital. It stopped when I went back to my job. I used to have hot flashes only at night but for the last two years I have them day and night. My doctor gave me hormones but they didn't help. It's very hard to be close to people at work when it happens as I feel like I stink. It happens at least 4 or 5 times a day and at night. I wake up at least 3 or 4 times wet and sweaty and then take off the covers and fall asleep and wake up again because I'm cold.

Truthfully I have experienced very little change because of menopause. My energy level is less. Sexually I did not have

much desire before so it hasn't changed. I have very little
desire now. Flashes that I got only lasted six months. The
nights were the worst time for this but I did not ever take
anything during the change. I had had no depression. I
think being physically active all my life helps during meno-
pause. Your outlook on life means much and [because of]
this [menopause] has not made any difference to me. I
started my change five years ago and if it were not that my
period stopped I would never know of a change (besides the
six months of hot flashes).

Menopause is experienced by more women today than ever
before. Had you been born two hundred years ago, you probably
would not have lived much past your childbearing years and,
therefore, would not have reached a menopause. Until recently
a woman's life span was usually shorter than her reproductive
capacity—most women died before reaching menopause. But
today, especially with informed self-care, a woman can expect to
live thirty or forty vigorous years *after* the first signs of menopause
appear. This book is planned to help women understand the
process they will go through during those years, how unpleasant
some of the symptoms can be, and what women can do about
them.

As a woman, you are in a unique position today. Investigators
are now publishing studies that show how hormone alterations,
hormone replacement therapy, diet, and sexual behavior all influence the physical and mental processes of women. Until recently
it would not have been possible to write a comprehensive book
on menopause—not enough was known. But now enough is
known. There is an abundance of new information which can be
found in many research articles. Each describes a small but critical
aspect of menopausal physiology. Now is the time to assemble this
information.

Normally, it takes five to six years for the knowledge of new biomedical discoveries to reach the public. First it takes two years for the results of a research study to be published in the scientific journals. The two years from completion of a study is followed by another two years before scholarly review articles appear that can incorporate the findings into their summaries. It is through such predigested review articles that the time-pressured professionals often try to keep abreast of recent advances. A year or two later the information may finally trickle down to you.

The problem of timing is not so critical from an intellectual and historical viewpoint. But for you, a woman going through menopause, a five- or six-year delay in obtaining information that may help you to enhance your life can be unfortunate. With this book it may be possible for you to circumvent the usual five-year delay. It should serve as a basic reference for you, even as new discoveries continue to be made.

To the consternation of many women, some health professionals have hinted that menopause problems are really a mental (neurotic) condition without basis in physiology. This is more a reflection of an insensitivity to the complex physiology of women than it is to any "fact" of neurosis. Menopausal distress is real. While many subtleties remain unexplained, it has been repeatedly shown that hormone levels have certain clear-cut and simple correspondences both with distress and with freedom from distress.

The issues involved in menopausal health care are complex. And the answers are often not simple. For example, you might ask: Should I use hormone therapy to treat my hot flashes? If yes, then how much hormone is "safe," and for what period of time should it be taken? If you do take hormones that have been prescribed for you and your breasts become sore, you might wonder: Am I taking too high a dosage?

A great deal has been written about the menopause. As a layperson, how can you separate fact from fancy when you read sensational claims in the newspapers and in new books? As a layperson, how do you decide whether to believe those who tell you that hormone replacement therapy is the fountain of youth or those who tell you that it is a deadly and unnecessary evil? Some women take vitamin E. As a layperson, how do you decide whether vitamin E treatment will improve your well-being or waste your money?

One answer is to become alert to the biases inherent in much media reporting. Be suspicious of news that presents only one side of an issue and the data that support only one particular perspective. Because a good reporter knows that he or she, as a nonscientist, is incapable of reaching technical/scientific conclusions, good reporting presents all sides. A sophisticated reader can usually identify biased reports by recognizing their sensational approach to their topics. If you read that hormone replacement therapy is an elixir of youth and are then provided only with the series of studies proving this, be on your guard. If you read that hormone replacement therapy is an evil thing that has been perpetrated upon innocent women and do not read anything positive about it, again be on your guard. Remember, there are no simple answers to the complex issues of the maturing years.

Once you are alert to the biases, you should develop a health maintenance plan that will most effectively serve your needs through your menopause. To do this requires that you get in tune with your body. You need to learn how to listen to what it tells you in order to enjoy it and to make changes when it is hurting.

You will need the strength of will to secure the type of health care which *you* decide is best for *you*. To do this may require that you overcome old habits of placing responsibility for yourself in the hands of others. To maximize your health, you must take responsibility for yourself because only *you* can know how you feel. Only you are experiencing your body's pains. Only you are feeling its well-being.

In this era of prolonged extension of life, eighty-five years is a common span while menopause usually begins in the mid-forties. You have a lot of years to live after the onset of menopause. It's important to plan for them. To do this you need the facts. In order to prepare this book, thousands of research reports have been evaluated and cross-checked to bring you these facts. In this book you will also find the comments of women who are currently being studied at Stanford as well as those of women from the Philadelphia area. The perspective provided by these women combined with a separate analysis of the relevant biomedical literature bring an unusually broad focus to this text.

This book is the story of the menopause. As the chapters unfold it will describe how

- beginning at around age forty-three (seven years before the last menstrual flow) menstrual cycle lengths and bleeding quantities change and symptoms usually begin. This is due to the aging and shrinking of the ovaries and the consequent decline in blood levels of estrogen and other hormones.

- the symptoms are experienced in varying degrees of severity by about 85 percent of women. Hot flashes, night sweats, insomnia, and a loss of a sense of well-being are common. In addition, for about 50 percent of women a progressive loss of bone begins which, if unchecked, produces the disease called osteoporosis.

- after menses stop, hormonal levels continue to decline and symptoms may persist for many years.

Following hormones and symptoms, we will then discuss

- how the body's changes in response to hormonal signals include changes in skin, vagina, urinary tract, breast, bone-calcium content, and possibly memory.

the critical changes that bones undergo as estrogen levels decline, as well as the effects of these changes on general health.

Having considered these basics, we next focus on hormone replacement therapy, which may help certain problems but, due to its inherent nature, may create others.

Next, we will consider your sexuality in the face of your own and your partner's changes.

Then menopausal surgery is discussed. This includes hysterectomy, the operation that is performed on approximately half of all women. We will take up its benefits, risks, side effects, and the arguments for retaining your ovaries even if you agree that your uterus should be removed.

And then, for those who want more physiological detail, three appendices are given, which review, in detail, the research facts, and figures to support the claims made in this book. They also provide you with guidelines of dosages for certain vitamins and minerals that you may decide to incorporate into your plan.

Finally, a checklist is provided at the end of the book to guide you in reviewing the details of your own health care.

At one time, the doctor assumed all the responsibility for a woman's health care. The woman was docile and evinced the unquestioning faith she had in her doctor, probably the most critical factor in promoting health care. Once upon a time you may have believed that a doctor could cure your ills and optimize your well-being. Were you taught, as a child, that when you were ill (or to maintain your health) your ultimate resource was your doctor? Were you lucky enough to have a doctor who provided the warmth and kindness to cause you to believe this? And how about today? When you seek gynecological help with vaginal dryness, or hot flashes, or menopausally related loss of the sense of well-being, or any other legitimate menopausal complaint, does your doctor provide real help?

Modern science and the pressures of society have created a different attitude toward the health-care field today, yet the illusion of the old-fashioned doctor often persists. It still is long, arduous, and costly to become a physician. However, in most other respects the medical profession has changed. Today, for each opening in medical school, there are at least three outstanding candidates. Lawsuits have been brought and won which insure that entry to medical schools will be based on the objective criteria of excellent academic performance rather than the independent judgment of the admissions committees. Because of this fierce competition and resulting emphasis on academic standing, qualities of humanity, gentleness, patience, and empathy are often not given sufficient consideration in selecting our nation's future doctors. What we have gained in objectivity we may have lost in subjectivity—that is, in our doctors' ability and willingness to offer concerned and kind care. We shouldn't necessarily blame the doctor. The young man or woman who starts out wanting to serve others by becoming a physician very soon learns that the *only* way he or she will have a chance of occupying a seat in medical school is to develop a single-minded pursuit of the highest possible test scores in college. Only the strongest can make it.

We have taught these students as undergraduates and at medical school. They are bright, intelligent, articulate, and hard-working. The system requires them to become self-centered enough to earn very high grades; to do so they must usually enter into severe competition with their classmates. University faculties can be irritated by the hard-driving premed students, but their pique often seems to reinforce a student's idea that he or she must either compete vigorously or else give up the dream of medical school. Those who do manage to be accepted into medical school face another four pressure-filled years in which they must learn to think fast, respond instantly, and repress their natural sensitivities to the large number of often painful human problems with which they are confronted on a daily basis. Those who go on to specialize in gynecology (an obstetrical-surgical subspecialty) must go through further training for several more years (the years vary depending on the specialty) in which they must rapidly digest enormous amounts of information. It is little wonder that the training process often teaches the doctors to rush, to ignore their own (and others) feelings, to lack compassion, and in general to be more concerned about plowing through and completing their enormous work load than about being reflective and displaying gentleness. The demands on the physician's time and energy— including the needs of patients, and the necessity of keeping abreast of a constantly expanding body of medical knowledge and alert to the possibilities of malpractice suits—aggravate and intensify the pressures.

One way this is reflected is when doctors make their own time a priority while showing no respect for the value of their patient's time. It is common to see a waiting room filled with patients who have all been scheduled for 9:00 A.M. appointments and who will be seen throughout the course of the next four hours. Fortunately, not all practicioners are so inconsiderate. In fact, the truly caring physician is just as likely to have a full waiting room, but for a very different reason. On occasion your problem may take more time than the scheduled time allotted. If the doctor cares about you, he or she will, to provide good medical care, take whatever time you need. This may cause other patients to be delayed. Many physicians only delay patients when an unavoidable situation (an emergency or extra patient needs) occur. The critical question is: Why are you delayed? The answer can guide your decision about your choice of health-care professional.

Many doctors are very well informed scientifically. Often they know the latest research on risks and benefits of particular treatments. *Take advantage of the times in which we live. There has never been a better time for a woman to maximize her health care.* Make use of what is available to you: (1) the knowledge of a physician who keeps himself or herself up to date; (2) a book like this one that can be a good personal resource volume; and (3) a strong sense of your self-worth (which requires giving up your emotional and intellectual dependency on the medical establishment). Then you can reap a rich harvest in health care. If you focus your energy on learning about your body and searching for a competent physician who will respect and work with you, you can enjoy a level of health unknown to previous generations.

Don't be afraid to ask questions of your doctor. Make a list of questions before you see him or her. Mailing a copy to your doctor before your appointment may be a good idea. Write down his or her answers to your queries. These notes will give you something to study when you get home; study is probably necessary if you are not a scientist because much of the communication problem between doctors and their patients results from the use of a technical vocabulary. Although your doctor is probably busy and he or she is entitled to your consideration when it comes to his or her time, you also have legitimate rights. You are paying for your doctor's services and are entitled to assurance that you have understood his or her comments. Very often, your physician's knowledge and terminology is beyond your usual understanding. By writing down what your doctor says and checking with him or her for accuracy, you can reread what you have written later and make sure that you have completely understood what he or she has told you. Remember, others are waiting for a turn. If you are well prepared and your questions are to the point, a good physician, in a minimal amount of time, will be happy to assure you that you have understood him or her.

This book provides the tools needed to help you work with a physician. You may be fortunate in that your health habits and hormone levels are adequate to maintain vibrant health. Good! More likely, however, you are having some of the symptoms of menopause that were described earlier. To alleviate these symptoms, you may want to seriously consider hormone therapy. It is important to realize that the recent proliferation of medical malpractice suits has put physicians in the unfortunate position of being defensive about the treatments they are willing to suggest. In many cases, a woman has to *ask* for hormone replacement therapy in order to receive it—not because hormone replacement therapy is bad, but because the beleaguered medical community sometimes tends to feel there is less risk of problems by avoiding any risk.

It requires desire, will power, and time to become educated. But there are great rewards. Let us begin!

1 / The Sex Hormones

Menopause is the natural result of age-related changes in ovarian function. It means, literally, the cessation of uterine menstrual cycles. When two years have passed without a menstrual period, you can be 98-percent sure no more will ensue. To understand the menopause and the change of life that precedes it, you ought to know about hormones, where they are produced, and how they act. Hormones are very powerful substances. Minute concentrations of them will produce enormous effects on both your body and on your brain.

What are hormones?

Hormones are substances that travel in the blood. The blood that circulates through your body is much like a pot full of gravy.

Santo V. Nicosia, M.D., M.S. (Pathology, Associate Professor of Obstetrics and Gynecology, and Pathology), Hospital of the University of Pennsylvania, has generously given of his self and his knowledge, and has contributed the illustrative material on ovaries in this chapter.

If, when the gravy is simmering, you add water to it and stir it thoroughly, each spoonful will have about the same flavor and content as any other spoonful. Since the blood is continuously recirculating through your body, your heart's pumping action acts like a spoon, mixing and stirring the ingredients. Your glands produce hormones which are released into your blood stream. Your kidneys and digestive tract control the amount of water added to your blood. And, like gravy in the pot, the blood's ingredients blend and change form as they heat up and are mixed.

Hormones are substances that are produced in parts of the body called glands. They are tiny enough to travel in the blood to other parts of the body to exert their action. A hormone is like an itinerant preacher who travels about, influencing others wherever he goes. The blood serves hormones somewhat like the vehicle that transports the preacher. Blood travels everywhere in the body (within the arteries, capillaries, and veins), and the hormones in blood leave the blood stream when they reach a receptive tissue. The hormones that are most important in understanding the menopause are estrogen and progesterone. These are produced predominantly in the ovaries. An understanding of menopause, therefore, requires an understanding of the ovaries.

The ovaries

The ovaries of a woman may be the most remarkable structures in nature. Nowhere else in the human body, male or female, does an organ undergo a monthly cycle in which both the size and the content change from day to day in a regular and repeating pattern. In addition to this repeating monthly pattern, the ovaries change throughout life, too.

In the prepubescent girl the ovaries are small but already have all the eggs that she will ovulate over her entire lifetime. She is born with her lifetime supply of eggs and will never produce an additional one. Around each egg (ovum) lies a flat sheet of cells.

The entire structure of the egg with its covering sheet of cells is known as a follicle. (Plate A shows a magnified slice of a baby girl's ovary. Hundreds of follicles appear in this slice.

Since you are probably looking at a photograph of an electron micrograph for the first time, it is helpful to consider the perspective of the picture. First, a slice is taken from the ovary much as you might slice up a candy Easter egg. This slice is laid on a flat surface, and a piece of the slice is cut out much like you might use a cookie cutter to cut out sections of rolled dough when preparing to bake. All of the photographs in this chapter are mounted on small glass slides that are rectangular in shape. So when you look at the picture and see a very straight edge, this is the edge formed by the cut from the tissue sample before the ovarian slice was mounted. The ovary, itself, has no straight edges. Some of the pictures show a curving edge on one or more sides. In that case, you are probably looking at one of the outside edges of the ovary. Much like in the cookie-cutting analogy, you might sometimes cut out a cookie on the edge of the rolled-out dough and, in doing so, fail to get a cookie that is the same shape as the cutter.

The ovarian cycle

After puberty (usually around age twelve or thirteen, when pregnancy becomes possible) eight to ten of these follicles begin to mature each month. The cells of the follicular sheet multiply and fill with fluid. These follicular cells start to swell as the fluid laden with cholesterol enters them from the surrounding medium of the ovary. After the cholesterol is absorbed into the follicle, it is converted into the steroid hormones (predominantly estrogen), and some of these hormones leak back out of the follicle into the ovary. This leaked estrogen works its way into the blood vessels that lie nearby the follicle and gets carried out into the rest of the body through the blood stream. Usually, only one of each

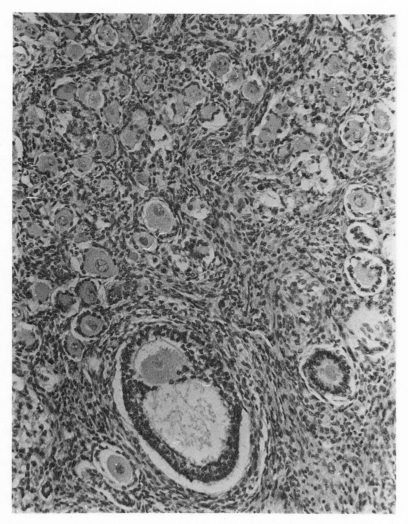

Plate A.   *Electron Micrograph of a Slice of an Ovary of a Baby Girl*

This magnified picture of a thin slice of ovary shows how some of the cells of the ovary collect into circular groupings called follicles. At the center of each follicle lies a single egg. Note in this picture the one big follicle and the many smaller ones. This picture does not show any of the outside edges of the ovary, just the more central region.

month's crop of follicles matures. The rest die. The one maturing follicle, then, keeps growing until it reaches its time of ovulation. "Ovulation" is the term that describes the release of the egg from its follicle and its escape from the outer surface of the ovary into the Fallopian tubes. As an egg begins its journey down the Fallopian tube (also called the oviduct) toward the uterus, the egg is available for a rendezvous with a penetrating sperm; if the egg is fertilized by sperm from the male, a pregnancy will usually result. Figure 1 shows where the ovaries and the uterus are located.

Each month, after ovulation, the cells that had formed the ruptured follicle, reconnect to each other and continue to multiply, swell, and take on a yellowish appearance. What was a follicle now becomes known as a corpus luteum (Latin for "yellow body"). The corpus luteum gets so large—by about seven days after ovulation—that it can take up half of the ovary, crowding the tiny follicles into the edges of the swelling ovary. The corpus luteum secretes estrogen and another hormone—progesterone. As the corpus luteum continues its growth, estrogen and progesterone levels in blood continue to rise. When the corpus luteum is at its largest, the progesterone level is at its highest—about seven days after ovulation. Then the corpus luteum begins a process of regression, shrinking in size as its cells die. Simultaneously, progesterone and estrogen levels in the blood decline. This "luteal regression" continues until the next menstruation occurs and the ovary is back once again to its smaller menstrual-phase size.

This ovarian cycle of follicle swelling, ovulation, corpus-luteum swelling, and shrinking repeats in a more or less regular monthly fashion until menopause. Even if the complexity of the ovarian cycle is new to you, the fact of your repeated menstrual cycle is not. Menstrual flows occur for a period of several days during each month. The flow is called "menstruation" after the Latin word menses, month. By scientific convention, the days of a woman's

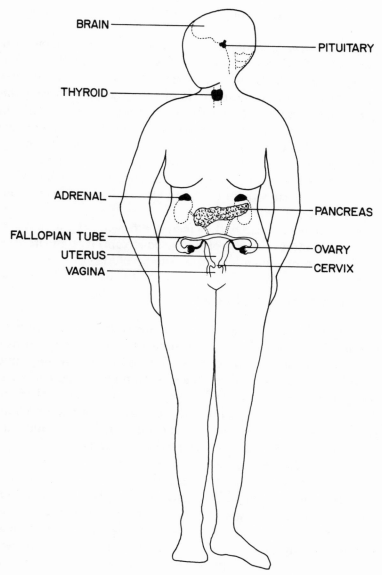

Figure 1 Female Reproductive Anatomy: Endo-crine Glands and Sexual Organs

menstrual cycle are counted from the first day of menstrual flow. "Day 1" stands for the first day of menstrual flow, "Day 10" stands for the day nine days after the menstrual onset, and so on. It is during the early days of the cycle that those eight to ten immature follicles in the ovary begin to swell. Plate B shows a magnified slice of ovary from a woman in her thirties. A number of developing follicles can be seen (look at the neatly circular structures). Plate C is a magnification of the largest follicle from the ovarian slice of the thirty-year-old woman. One can see a circular structure toward its center—the ovum (the egg).

As the follicles enlarge, they secrete estrogen. As the estrogen reaches the uterus (by way of the blood stream) it stimulates the development of the endometrium of the uterus.

The endometrial cycle

The endometrium is the layer of tissue that lines the inside of the uterus; it is a composite of glandular (secreting) tissue mixed with blood vessels and other cells. During the preovulatory time of the cycle, endometrial cells increase in number, the endometrial glands grow in size, and blood vessels grow in to them to provide nourishment. As a result, the thickness of endometrium greatly increases. These changes in endometrial composition are shown in the menstrual-cycle chart (Figure 2). This chart shows other cyclic changes (in the ovary, blood, etc.) as well. After the follicle has ovulated its egg the newly formed corpus luteum secretes both estrogen and progesterone. These two ovarian hormones produce even greater growth of the endometrium and endometrial blood supply. If, by fourteen days after ovulation, a fertilization has not occurred, the corpus luteum in the ovary will die. Without a corpus luteum, estrogen and progesterone levels drop drastically. This sudden withdrawal of hormonal support is followed by a rapid deterioration of the blood vessels in the

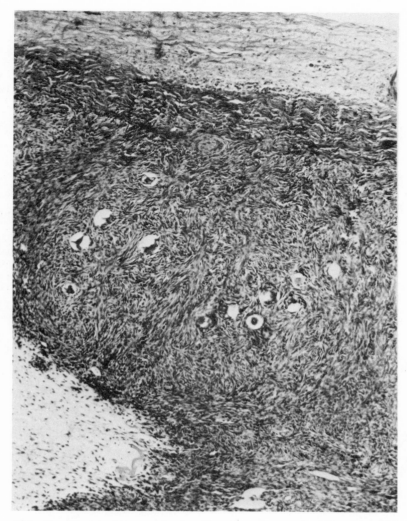

Plate B. *Electron Micrograph of a Slice of an Ovary of a Thirty-Year-Old Woman*

This magnified slice of an ovary from a woman in her thirties shows, at the top, the outer edge (cortex) of the ovary and also part of the more central region below. It also shows some small follicles that are developing.

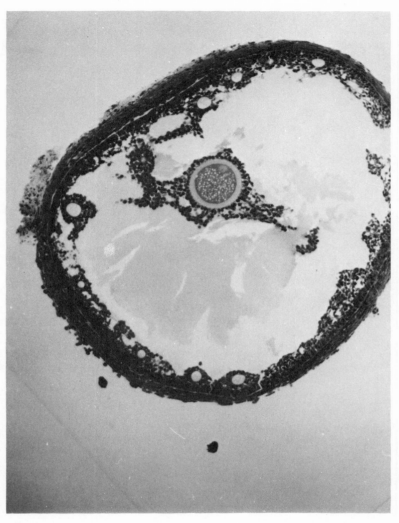

Plate C. *Electron Micrograph of a Slice of One Ovulatory Follicle from Plate B*

This picture shows one follicle that is very large and almost ready to ovulate. The circular structure toward the center is the egg that will leave the follicle and the ovary, and enter the Fallopian tube.

endometrium. The living cells die without blood to nourish them with oxygen. These dead cells from the endometrial tissue, along with blood and some mucus, form the menstrual fluid which leaves the body through the vagina. The bleeding soon stops, and the endometrial cycle begins anew.

The term "the change of life" describes a new pattern. At about age forty-three the ovaries begin their slow and gradual approach toward menopause. By menopause the ovary's supply of eggs is almost depleted, although a few may still remain. Developmental processes are beautifully synchronized in nature. It takes about seven years from the first menstrual period until a woman is fully fertile, and it takes about seven years for the reverse process (total infertility) to be complete. During this time the ovaries are gradually losing their ability to ovulate a follicle. The cycle of follicle swelling continues to occur, but the ovulation and subsequent corpus-luteum development increasingly fail to occur. Without an ovulation, there cannot be a conception. Pregnancy, after unprotected intercourse, becomes rarer, as women move through their forties and have fewer ovulatory cycles.

Exactly why the menopause occurs when it does is probably related to the gradual loss of eggs throughout life. But other factors must also interact because some few eggs do remain even after menstrual flows have ceased. Several other, seemingly unrelated pieces of information are also known, and many investigators are trying to figure out the rest of the puzzle. Surprisingly, there is no clear relationship between the age at which a woman has her first menstrual period and her age at menopause.[2, 17] Mothers of twins begin menopause about a year earlier than other mothers,[21] but why this is true is not yet understood. In addition, a woman who smokes is likely to begin menopause sooner than one who does not, and the more smoking she does, the sooner it will happen.[3, 8] We do not yet know how it happens, but it does appear that smoking affects your reproductive system.

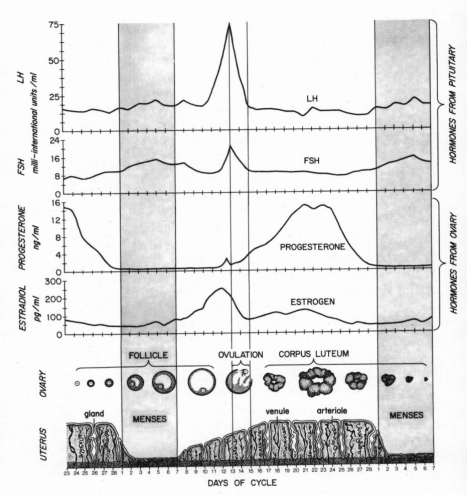

Figure 2 The Reproductive Cycle of Women: The Changes in Hormones, Ovarian Tissue, and Endometrium

How hormones change

As your ovary ages, its follicular tissue content decreases and with this the luteal phase level of estrogen and progesterone also decreases.[13, 15, 16] Since the corpus luteum is the main source (after ovulation each month) of both progesterone and estrogen, the severe decline in the levels of these hormones in the blood is inevitable. By the time menopause has occurred, clear changes in the ovaries are evident. For one thing, they have become smaller. Only a few follicles remain, but you can see in their place large masses of undifferentiated tissue called "stroma" as well as scattered follicle and corpus-luteum residues that look degenerated. You can see how different the ovary of a menopausal woman looks (Plate D) by comparing it with an ovary of a baby girl (Plate E). The pictures are magnified several hundred times so that you can see the actual follicular sheet described earlier.

But just because the menopausal ovary no longer ovulates each month, this does not mean that it has stopped working altogether. In fact, the central region of the ovary is filled with some healthy and very active cells that are making hormones. This region continues to work as a busy factory producing two androgens—

This chart (facing page) shows what is happening in different places at different times of the monthly cycle. For example, select day 2 of the cycle (see bottom line). Then look up in a straight line to see all the things recorded for day 2. (1) The uterus is menstruating, and the lining of the womb is, therefore, thinner than on any other day of the month. (2) The ovary contains a swelling follicle, sketched to show the tiny egg that the follicular cells surround. (3) The blood levels of hormones from the ovary are shown: first estrogen, then progesterone. Both are at relatively low levels compared to how high the levels of each will become on other days of the cycle. (4) Blood levels of the reproductive hormones produced in the pituitary are also shown. On day 2 of the cycle, for example, both follicle stimulating hormone (FSH) and luteinizing hormone (LH) are rising. Note that the units in which hormones are measured (picograms per milliliter of blood, nanograms per, or milli-international units) may be unfamiliar. The essential point is to notice how the levels change from day to day until one cycle is complete. Then the levels repeat that cycle to form the rhythmic ebb and flow of hormone concentration that circulate in the blood.

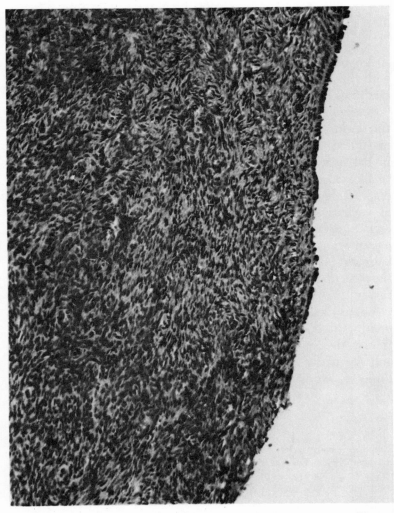

Plate D. *Electron Micrograph of a Slice of an Ovary of a Menopausal Woman*

This magnified slice of a menopausal ovary shows a part of the edge of the ovary along the right side. The straight edge at the top, bottom, and left side was formed from the edges of the glass slide on which the ovarian slice was mounted. Note the absence of large follicles.

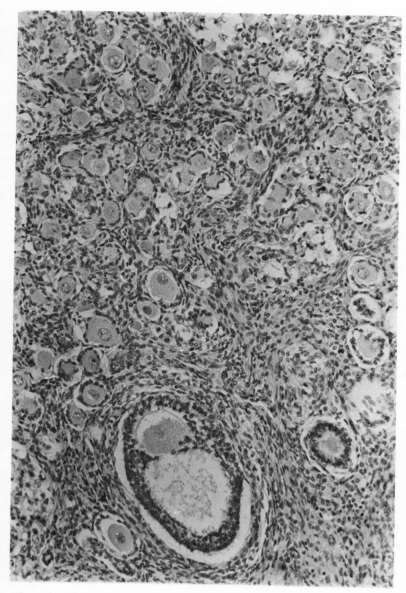

Plate E. *Electron Micrograph of a Slice of an Ovary of a Baby Girl*

androstenedione and testosterone—and delivers them into the blood stream.[1, 10, 11, 14] The word "androgen" is derived from the Greek *andro* for "masculine." Androstenedione and testosterone are the "male sex hormones," but women have them too although in much lesser quantities than do men. Older ovaries often produce more testosterone than younger ones,[9] which probably accounts for the mustache so commonly found in older women.

Just because the ovaries decrease their production of estrogen does not mean that you don't have any female hormones. The cells of fat you have now play a major role in your body's hormonal milieu. The more fat you have, the more estrogen you will have.[20, 19] A fat cell acts as a miniature factory. It takes up the androstenedione and converts it to estrone—a weak estrogen. The estrone gets converted further, possibly by cells in the liver, into molecules of estradiol. After menopause, the major source of estrone is supplied this way.[5, 6, 7, 10] This hormone, and the other hormones, are, among other things, important for well-being, bone health, skin suppleness, and prevention of heart disease. The overall estrogen levels vary enormously among menopausal women.[12] Some women have much higher levels than other women.

The adrenal glands

The ovaries aren't the only glands that produce hormones. The adrenal glands (there are two of them, each one resting on top of one of the two kidneys) produce a variety of hormones including cortisol, androgens, and small amounts of estrogens and progesterone. You can locate the adrenal glands by looking at Figure 1 (page 43). Both before and after menopause, the adrenal glands contribute small amounts of estrogen to your blood[18] as well as larger amounts of androstenedione and testosterone. But the adrenal glands also change with age, and around age fifty to fifty-five they decrease their output of androgen. "Adrenopause" is the term coined to describe this phenomenon.[4]

Summary

All of this may seem complicated, and it is. Here are the essentials. Sometime during a woman's forties, menstrual cycles become more irregular and eventually cease altogether. Menopause refers to the permanent cessation of menstrual cycles and is the natural result of age-related changes in ovarian function. Another consequence of this change in the ovaries is that the blood levels of estrogen are reduced by about 75 percent—an enormous reduction that can produce a tremendous shock to your body. It is important to understand that the decrease in estrogen occurs at precisely the time that menopausal problems begin. Menopausal symptoms appear to be caused by the body's desperate reaction to its sudden loss of hormonal support. In the next chapter a complete description of these symptoms is presented as well as a description showing why the time of menopausal transition is often called "the change of life."

2 / The Change
of Life

I am experiencing hot flashes almost every day. When I do get a period, it seems to take everything out of me. I am beginning to have difficulty coping with people. I find I get my feelings hurt easily. I'm avoiding certain jobs, responsibilities, because I just don't feel like I can handle them well. Sexual activity is infrequent [and] I find myself thinking of it less and less. Never seems to fit into my schedule. Roughly one week before I start a period, I get either terribly irritated at everyone and everything or extremely sensitive and feel like weeping over nothing. I never had the high ups and such low-downs as I have now.

I really haven't had too much discomfort physically but emotionally I have become more and more depressed. It's amazing how much better I feel after I get my period. I feel young again. Maybe I'm afraid of getting old.

I am delighted to no longer have menstrual periods as I always had painful ones—even within 3 periods of the birth of a baby. I am also very happy to have the remote possibility of pregnancy gone from my life. Since I had had the operation [mastectomy] I was never given any hormones and don't feel that I ever needed them. I was given meprobamate as a tranquilizer from my surgery in 1969 till lately. I have stopped refilling the prescription on my own because I feel I can get along just fine with nothing.

I have a general feeling of being old and fat and middle-aged —low self-image.

The change

The term "change of life" refers to a process of biological change in a woman's body that takes place over a span of about seven years.[11, 20, 24, 35, 40, 41] It is during this time that her menstrual cycles become increasingly irregular, and it is at the end of this time, usually at around the age of fifty, that menopause begins.[25, 40, 41, 42, 43, 44] Naturally, these menstrual changes vary from woman to woman. Some women experience more frequent menstrual cycles than they had before this change began. Menstruation every twenty days or so is not uncommon. Others menstruate much less frequently, even as rarely as once a year.[42] Some women experience no change in cycle length but find that their flow pattern is different than it had been. You might find that the number of days or the amount of your flow has diminished, or that either or both have increased. Mixed patterns are also common. You might, for example, experience shorter cycles of heavier bleeding or infrequent menses with many days of very light flow. Just as likely, you might have a short cycle followed by a long one, and continued unpredictable cycles for several years. The point is that there are no fixed patterns of change to expect. There are wide varieties of changes possible, and they are normal to healthy women.

The time during which your cycle is changing but before you have reached menopause is called the "premenopause" or the "perimenopause." The Stanford Menopause Study, mentioned earlier in this book, began with normal, healthy, perimenopausal women. About 20 percent of them found that their menstrual flow had become so heavy or so continuous that dressing fastidiously became difficult for them. If you have these kinds of bleeding problems, it makes sense to seek help from your doctor. But even if your doctor examines you and says "You are okay—there is no disease—you are just approaching menopause," that does not make your problem any easier. Excessive bleeding weakens your system and can leave you feeling fatigued and lethargic. The important point for you to remember is that if you are experiencing long and heavy or erratic bleeding, you can get relief through proper medical management.[13] This will usually involve getting some progesterone, either by injection or pill. Ask your doctor about this. It is certainly worth the time to correct the problem.

If you were premenopausal and experiencing fairly regular menstrual cycles, your estrogen, progesterone, and testosterone levels would be constantly changing from day to day in a predictable and orderly rhythm. The ebb and flow of reproductive hormones during the cycling years is like a well-orchestrated symphony and equally as elegant. But as you enter your menopausal transition years, the new and irregular pattern of menstrual cycling reflects major upheavals in your hormonal milieu, caused at least in part by the decreasing presence of estrogens in your body. Your body is likely to respond to this decrease in a number of ways that generally cause a predictable pattern of physical and emotional distress.[34] These discomforts comprise the symptoms associated with both the perimenopause and the menopause. While many of these discomforts disappear several years after the last menstrual period, the experience of them can be especially unsettling if you do not know what to expect.

The symptoms of menopause

Hot flashes

What happens during a hot flash? In 1975 actual measurements were recorded.[26] A menopausal woman lay nude on a nylon net bed and was connected to various instruments which monitored her physiological changes. Each flash lasted about 3½ minutes. During the flash there was a sudden rise of about one to four degrees Farenheit in her skin temperature. At the beginning of the flash her heart would suddenly beat much faster, but as the flash progressed her heart rate returned to normal. Any time the brain perceives that the body is overheated, whether from fever or any other source, a series of reflex changes in blood flow predictably causes the body to attempt to relieve its heat. Blood vessels near the skin dilate and blood pours into this path bringing heat to the skin. The heat radiates out to the skin. The heated skin begins to perspire, and evaporation cools things down. So it is with the hot flash. The brain gets a sudden signal that the body is too hot. We do not yet know what triggers the hot-flash signal since there is no fever, but the reflex response just described occurs anyway. For the woman who's case study is being detailed, each time a flash started, she reported a sudden shock of intense heat. She showed a rapidly accelerating heartbeat and sweat profusely on her forehead and nose, moderately on her chest and adjacent regions, but not at all on her cheeks. Her water loss from each flash episode was about one teaspoon. These changes in temperature were widespread throughout her body. In fact, even the finger and toe temperatures showed a sharp rise at the beginning of a flash. Then they returned to normal several minutes after the flash had ended. This woman's reaction is not unique. Other investigators have reported the same general pattern in their studies.

Hot flashes are flashes of heat that, at first, can be an alarming experience. The body suddenly feels intensely hot. About three minutes later the flash is gone. Here are some descriptions from women that have experienced them.

Since reaching menopause, I have experienced frequent hot flashes where it even seems as though I could feel much more comfortable without my skin.

I perspire profusely with perspiration running down my face and my back. It lasts for a few minutes and then I feel chilled.

Occasional hot flash—feel like a boiled tomato with skin ready to burst—mild perspiration.

The hot flashes are very intense but of short duration. It is mostly my head that feels very hot. Sometimes my ears and my face get red. There also seems to be an increase in pressure in my head at that time. The hot flashes come frequently when I have them but there are long stretches of time when I do not have any. While they are very uncomfortable, except for my fear that other people will notice that my face is getting red, they have not interfered with my life at all.

I always claimed that my thermostat went crazy and even today I go from hot to cold and back again—a little uncomfortable but nothing I cannot live with. A minimum dosage of estrogen has been prescribed.

Hot flashes are experienced by more than 85 percent of women going through menopause, although there is a wide variation in how often they come and how hard they hit.[2, 10, 22, 37] For some, only a few mild flashes each week or so will occur. For others (25 percent to 50 percent) flashes can be very troublesome even ten years after the last menstrual period.[4, 18, 33] In severe cases hot flashes may come as often as six or seven times every hour, and this pattern can last for many years. For two out of three women hot flashes start well before the last menstruation arrives.[37] Generally, the flashes increase dramatically at menopause and continue to occur, with intermittent flash-free periods (sometimes lasting several months), for about the next five years.[1] When a woman first begins to experience flashing, the flushes are infrequent and are felt on the face and neck only. Once they start, they tend to get worse before they get better.

Although hot flashes are not dangerous, they are uncomfortable. Moreover, it is a special kind of discomfort that is not the same as being simply overheated. One group of investigators used hot water bottles and blankets in order to learn whether they could induce hot flashes in premenopausal women by making them very warm. They couldn't. Even when premenopausal women are heated up by external means, they do not show the change in heart rate and blood pressure typical of a menopausal hot flush.[35]

Hot flashes, though, are aggravated by hot weather.[27] While hot summer weather probably won't cause hot flashes, it may contribute to your distress if you are having periods of flushing. In one study of several menopausal women conducted during the months of June and July, hot flashes occurred more frequently on hotter days than on cooler days.[9]

We know that hot flashes are caused by a decrease in estrogen, because (1) flashes appear in association with the fall in estrogen that is characteristic of the change of life, and (2) they are eliminated when estrogen is taken. But why does a flash come when it does? What causes it? The onset of a hot flash corresponds to an increase in the blood level of a pituitary hormone called "luteinizing hormone" or LH for short.[7, 36] Significant changes in levels and rhythms of LH secretion are common as menopause nears[30] and appear to be one of the responses the body makes to the shrinking ovary's decrease of estrogen secretion. But other internal secretion surges also occur during hot flashes.[20] Furthermore, just after the flash other hormonal changes occur. For example, a significant rise in the blood level of some of the adrenal hormones (dehydroepiandrosterone, androstenedione, and cortisol) also occurs at this time.[24] Although there are clear relationships between hot flashes and specific hormone changes, the issues are complex[6] and we don't yet know whether or not these changes actually produce the flash.

Night sweats

About a year after I discontinued use of the [oral contraceptive] pill, I started mild menopause symptoms. For the next five years I went through the sudden hot flashes of the skin and the night sweats, etc. But the symptoms weren't consistent enough to alarm me.

Because of flashes up to about 2 months ago, my husband sleeps by himself—so I can have more comfort alone. It is impossible to sleep with anyone as I am wet over most of my body and have to open windows."

Night sweats appear to be the sleep-time equivalent of daytime hot flashes. If you have them, you will be waking up hot and drenched with sweat. Most women who experience night sweats also have daytime hot flashes, but the reverse doesn't always occur. That is, if you have hot flashes during the day, you won't necessarily have night sweats.[37] Night sweats can also be a symp-

tom of emotional distress that has nothing to do with the menopause. But if you begin to experience night sweats while you are
having daytime hot flashes, they are probably a part of your
change of life.

If you are perimenopausal (still cycling, though erratically) or
postmenopausal and find yourself waking in the night a great deal,
night sweats may be one reason for this. Sleeplessness in postmenopausal women has been studied and has always been found
to be closely linked with night sweats.[37] In the Stanford Menopause Study women described waking up after they had thrown
off their covers to relieve the intense heat of a flash. Often, they
had to get up to change their clothing and bed linen because one
or both would be drenched with sweat. The most severe cases
involved several changes each night.

If you are having a similar experience, you should be aware that
polyester and nylon (in nightclothes and bed linen) act like sheets
of plastic wrap holding the sweat next to your body, thus intensi-
fying your discomfort. Switching to pure cotton clothing and bed
linen should help you find some relief.

What can we conclude about hot flashes? The flash is a real
physiological process. An intense, feverlike heat comes suddenly,
lasts a minute or two or three, and then disappears. The heart
rhythm goes wild. The flash leaves in its wake a sweaty face and
chest. A flash is uncomfortable, and the accompanying skin flush
and sweating can be embarrassing. Sudden and intense sweating
in the middle of a business or social situation can be a disquieting
challenge to one's dignity. But a simple remedy does provide
rapid, though temporary, relief. Cooling yourself with a fan or
cold water splashed on your cheeks ends the flash faster.

A lot of women take vitamin E, thinking it might help. In fact
it doesn't, according to carefully controlled studies.[21, 16] What
does help, if cooling proves inadequate, is estrogen therapy in a
dosage sufficient to compensate for your newly changing ovarian
declines.[5, 8, 11] We will say more about this in Chapters 5 and 6.

Skin aging

Your skin ages more rapidly at menopause.[28, 29, 31, 32] As the estrogen level declines, the skin gradually loses both its thickness and some of its fluid. As a consequence, it rapidly begins to look older. Your sensitivity to the ultraviolet rays of the sun also increases as you grow older. This is because the number of tanning pigments (melanocytes) decreases the older you get.[23] Therefore, with the approach of the menopause you should take great care to avoid overexposure to the sun.

Loss of libido

A large proportion of perimenopausal and postmenopausal women apparently experience a decline in sexual interest.[19] In the Stanford Menopause Study, 71 percent of the women made comments about changes in their interest in sex since they had noticed changes in their menstrual cycles. Forty-eight percent reported a noticeable decline in sexual interest, and most were distressed about this. Twenty-three percent noticed an increase in libido. And 29 percent reported that interest in sex was unchanged. Therefore, regardless of your personal experience, a good number of women are experiencing things in pretty much the same way. We will discuss changing sexuality in Chapter 7.

Offensive menstrual odor

A number of the perimenopausal women in the Stanford Menopause Study described a problem they had that had never happened to them before—an offensive odor when they menstruated. Unfortunately, scientists do not know a great deal about this. The fluid of the vagina normally tends to be somewhat acidic, much the way vinegar or lemon juice is. The natural acid provides a hostile environment to most bacteria. Vaginal acidity does change as the estrogen levels decline,[29a] and without the high acid level to kill them odorous bacteria may begin to flourish in the vaginal tract. Trying an acidic remedy like one of the vaginal pH creams may be sufficient for most simple bacterial infections. More stubborn infections may require more specific aggressive treatment.

Memory loss

This issue has not been studied, but a great many of the Stanford women mentioned that they had recently noticed a memory-loss problem. They made comments like "I forget appointments," "Things which used to be easy to remember now take effort," "I forget where I put things." This could be due to hardening of the arteries, another problem that occurs in estrogen-deficient individuals. If this is happening to you, you might consider reducing the amount of fatty foods in your diet. This is a common-sense approach that can only enhance your health.

Visual deficits

This problem has also not been studied. Many women reported that with the change in their cycles, they had noticed changes in their visual abilities. They had trouble seeing road signs. They needed to change eyeglass prescriptions. Is the problem related to hormone changes at menopause? Only future studies can say.

Formication

Skin tingling or a feeling that unseen insects are crawling across your skin is called formication. It is a symptom of menopausal distress.[18, 21] A study of a group of 5,000 women revealed that the greatest incidence of formication happened within twelve to twenty-four months after the last menstrual period, when 20 percent of the menopausal women reported the problem. About 10 percent of women continued to be annoyed with the formication for more than the next twelve years, after the menopause. Eventually, it disappears. But its exact cause is still unknown.

Backache

Backache is common. Nonradiating pains (that is, the pain is localized and does not spread outward from the point of origin) begin at the lower back, and these may indicate the beginning of a loss in bone structure. This is a condition known as osteoporosis and is discussed in detail in Chapter 4.

Emotional distress

Sometimes I get a sort of "trembly" roller coaster ride feeling . . . just a trembly feeling like you'd have after the roller coaster ride. It's so hard to put into words, really. Fluttering; trembling; uneasy. Guess they could all be lumped under the heading of "anxiety." A vague uneasiness.

I have become more aggressive, more outspoken and assertive, less patient. I am easier on myself and less caring about what others think. Sexual activity has become much more enjoyable. My libido is increasing all the time and I look forward to sex. I don't seem to mind aging. I actually enjoy the maturing process.

Never had hot flashes, or other symptoms. Did undergo depression—for which I had to be treated—but doctors were unable to agree on whether or not it was the result of menopause or other factors at the time. My personal feeling is that I did suffer some kind of chemical imbalance which may have triggered depression. Extreme tension and stress since then have not produced another depression (thank God)!

I am often irritable and cranky without any good reason . . . cry often. I often feel very depressed for no reason at

*all and have very little energy. This all occurred very sel-
domly before.*

Of course, headache, depression, anxiety, listlessness, insomnia,
and backache also happen to women (and men, too!) who are not
menopausal. Still, the fact is that these things are experienced by
many menopausal women, and if you are experiencing them, it
may be useful to know that sleep disturbances do respond well to
estrogen therapy.[38, 39] The details are described in Chapter 5.

Who experiences menopausal distress?

Menopausal distress (the flashes, night sweats, libidinal
changes, etc.) hits both healthy and not so healthy women, and
your general level of health doesn't seem to have much to do with
whether you will suffer or escape from menopausal distress.[2]
However, some women are more at risk than others. Specifically, married women experience worse symptoms than single
women;[2, 18] those who have given birth have worse symptoms
than those who have not;[18] and those who experienced painful
menstruation when younger are more likely to experience
menopausal distress when older.[2] The facts are clear; at the mo-
ment the reasons are not yet understood.

Although some experts believe that women with menopausal
distress are neurotic, a careful and critical review of the literature
shows that menopausal distress is hormonally caused and hormonally cured. Yet some student health professionals are still exposed
to the following: "These symptoms are of sufficient magnitude in
approximately 15% of women to warrant treatment. If psychotherapy fails, daily administration of estrogen . . . will reverse the
symptoms."[15] Research shows psychotherapy to be irrelevant.
The hormones are the issue.

Several studies have explored large groups of women in search
of possible relationships among roles, behaviors, and a tendency

toward menopausal distress. The assumption underlying the questions has been that there must be a large psychological component in the perception of distress and that culturally accepted norms might actually be at the root of a woman's self-perception. The possibility that women in Western society reach menopause only to find an "empty nest" and suddenly empty days was considered by several investigators. They reasoned that roles which were forced on women had tended to keep them home raising children and keeping house.

Most of today's menopausal women have found themselves at the tail end of the women's movement. Even if they agree with its tenets of career rights for women, they may perceive thirty to forty years of housekeeping as an insurmountable obstacle toward major change in their lives. At this point, they may want a career but feel overwhelmed by difficulties such as a lack of career training or knowing how to handle an interview. In short, there can be a general feeling of incompetence due to lack of marketable skills.

Children often leave home or enter adolescence with all its difficulties at just about the time that many women are entering menopause. Could all the complaints of menopause be a simple reaction to a feeling that life has nothing further to offer? Is the reason that unmarried women have less distress simply that they have suffered no sudden loss of meaning coinciding with their menopause? Some health professionals thought so.

Pauline Bart, a well-respected social scientist, described depression problems in middle-aged women. She expressed her belief that our society has robbed women of a place of esteem at menopause.[3] You have only to look at the media, with its adoration of youth and beauty and its advertisements to "hide that gray" or camouflage wrinkles, to see her point.

If menopausal symptoms are the result of society's treatment of women, then we would expect to find no symptoms in those societies that revere their aging women and show this by affording them special privileges and honors. For example, the Hutterites (a culturally isolated sect of North America) automatically relieve the woman of her heavy jobs in agriculture when she reaches forty-five to fifty. They show an increased admiration for their maturing women, which is reflected in the older women's domination of their extended family.[17] Another well-characterized "primitive culture," the Quemant (a pagan Hebraic peasant group of Ethiopia), allows the menopausal woman the special privilege of treading upon normally taboo village sites. Furthermore, only after menopause does a woman reach sufficient status to be allowed to come in contact with ritual food and beverage.[14] Although both cultures revere their aging women, no study has ever evaluated menopausal distress in these societies.

Furthermore, in spite of studies designed to show cultural influences on menopausal symptoms, no proof has been offered. For example, a study appearing in *Psychosomatics*, a widely respected medical journal, has been extensively quoted, although the conclusions that were drawn appear to be misleading. Its author suggested that cultures which debase older women may actually create a "menopausal syndrome."[12] The article cited an extensive field study of 483 Indian women of one caste. No mention of hot flashes or other menopausal distress symptoms was made by any of them, which seemed to suggest to the author of the study that these women did not experience any. If it were true that hot flashes—the major symptom of menopause—are culturally induced, this would provide some extraordinary evidence for the influence of culture on individual hormone processes. However, our careful examination of the details of data collection showed that the research design itself had practically prohibited mention of hot flashes. Each woman in the study was asked a long series of questions about her marital, reproductive, and family history in the public circle of the women of her village. Only one question about menopause was asked, and this had nothing to do with hot flashes: "Any complications of menopause such as hysterectomy or prolapse?" This one question was embedded within a series of other questions which were concerned with nonmenopausal issues. Consider that only the very serious conditions of hysterectomy (surgical removal of the uterus) and prolapse (the dropping of the uterus into or out of the vagina) were mentioned. Even if a woman were suffering from hot flashes, this form of questioning might well have obscured that fact. Although this important study has been widely quoted, there is yet no real proof that flashes are a culturally induced pathology.

The idea that menopausal distress strikes the neurotic woman, while certainly possible, has never been truly proven. One investigator reported that there were no appreciable differences in personality traits among women who did and who did not have menopausal distress. Nor were there any detectable personality changes within individuals after successful hormone treatment. Neurosis and menopause troubles were not related. One can certainly imagine how real distress could cause a woman to seek medical help. If her "help" takes the form of insinuations that she is neurotic, it seems possible that she could begin to lose confidence in her own perceptions and thereby fulfill this diagnosis while still suffering the real distress associated with menopause. One woman at Stanford illustrated such a case:

Women on both sides of my family have had lots of atheroscelortic heart disease, manifesting itself at menopause. I'm concerned about this for reasons which I consider valid, but most doctors consider neurotic. In some ways, my stress EKG was borderline; i.e., very poor exercise tolerance for a woman of my age (44) and weight (slender)—yet I've been dealt with as a bored housewife (which I am not).

Summary

The "change of life" is a process that women go through as they approach and pass through their menopause. It has many manifestations. Menstrual cycles become more irregular and eventually cease altogether. This results from the aging of the ovaries. One critical result of a shrinking ovary is a decrease in the amount of estrogen in the body. When your menstrual cycles become irregular, the chances are strong that you will experience some of the symptoms described in this chapter.[7, 9, 11, 14, 19, 20, 22, 24, 35, 40, 41] Hot flashes and some degree of emotional distress are very common. Women tend to suffer alone. However, talking with others who have long since passed through their change of life is likely to be a reassuring experience. You will find that you are not alone and that eventually things do readjust for the better. Compare notes with other women. It should assure you of the realities of the menopause as well as help you to realize that relief is available.

3 / Body Changes at the Menopause

I feel that my body is changing but I really can't understand how it is or what is changing.

I had always heard that a shock sometimes stopped periods permanently and this happened to me. At 52, I was still having regular, normal periods although I started slowly the first day. This was happening when I got word my Mother had died. My period never developed and I never had another one.

The body is changing in a number of well-understood ways as the menopause approaches.

How skin ages

Remember, the estrogens decline at menopause and are likely to accelerate skin aging. So you need to take special care of your skin after age forty. There is beauty at every age, and since skin is one of the main surface reflections of your beauty, it makes sense to focus on this area first.

With increasing age a number of skin changes occur.[14] These include

- decreased tensile strength (that is ability to tense up)
- decreased compressibility and mobility
- decreased or general loss of turgor (firmness coming from water-filled cells)
- slight decreases in total skin collagen (one of the main supporting proteins)
- a continual loss of melanocytes (the cells that manufacture melanin, the pigment that causes your skin to tan)

One of the most important things you can do is to guard your skin from the damaging rays of the sun. As the years pass, you will be less protected from exposure to sunlight. This is because the number of melanocyte cells in your skin decreases by 10 percent to 15 percent each decade.[11] Sun screens are relatively new. Those that retard ultraviolet radiation are most helpful for maintaining the vigor and attractiveness of your skin. Since overexposure to sun is bad, the most prudent choice would appear, where possible, to limit your exposure. If you make a habit of avoiding sunbathing, or at least limiting it to the early and late hours of the day, you will reduce the intensity of your exposure to the aging effects of ultraviolet rays. The rays are less powerful when the sun is less bright.

When you think of skin, you may think of tissue that is on the outside of your body. Similar kinds of cells (epithelia) also line the urinary tract as well as the vagina. So, it is not surprising to find changes in both of these when skin starts to change.

Breast and abdominal changes

As women get older, their breasts tend to flatten and sag. The larger the breasts, the greater the tendency to flatten. There is a physiological reason for this.

Breast tissue responds to a good many hormones, including estrogens, prolactin, oxytocin, prostaglandins, and others. As the hormone levels change with the progression of the menopause, there is a withdrawal of the estrogen stimulation to all tissue, including the breast. As a consequence, the breasts begin to lose some of their earlier fullness. Women who take hormone therapy (see Chapters 6 and 7), however, will find some restoration of this fullness, with the response lasting for as long as hormones are available.

Because breast cancer is among the most common of the female cancers, it is very important that women examine their breasts regularly. Early detection of a cancerous tumor allows time for treatments that have a high success rate as well as a decreased likelihood of disfigurement.

The breasts should be examined in two ways: visually and by touch. The first is done by standing in front of a mirror in good light and looking for dissimilarities (not size but shape differences) between the two breasts. For example, flattening, puckering, dimpling of the skin, notable bulges, or any growths of the breast surface that appear suddenly in one breast would be cause for a medical examination. Having completed the visual inspection, the manual inspection (palpation) follows.

The breasts should be palpated periodically (about once a month). If being done by a premenopausal woman, the examination should occur immediately after the menstrual flow has stopped. Although some physicians suggest lying down, we feel it can also be done standing up. A sensible time is while you are showering or bathing. Because moist, soapy fingers can gently slide over the skin of the breast, compressing up and down and side to side, you will be able to feel whether there are any differences between the two breasts. Gently, you should tug the breasts away from the body with a gentle squeezing motion while you are using soapy and wet fingers. Do this on both sides and compare what is felt on one side to what is felt on the other feeling for lumpiness. These examinations should be done in two positions; with your hand at your side and with your arm elevated and your hand touching the back of your head. Do one breast and then the other in each of the two positions. These actions will place the breasts in position for efficient exploration. As long as they feel similar on both sides, there is no cause for concern.

It is important to know that lumpy breasts and breast pain are very common, occurring in about 35 percent of all women. These lumps (or cysts) usually do not have any relationship to breast cancer. Tumors can feel similar to these lumps, but an expert can distinguish which tissue should be tested and, from the test results, the healthy from the diseased tissue. If anything feels questionable, see your physician for expert advice. Even if you have recently had your breasts checked by your health-care provider, your self-examinations should continue every month. Films and literature on breast self-examination can be obtained by calling or writing the American Cancer Society, 777 Third Avenue, New York, New York 10017, 212–371–2900.

Women who exercise regularly should not notice changes in the size and shape of the abdomen. But women who have stopped having periods and who notice sudden increases in the size of their abdomen should be warned and make an appointment to see their gynecologist. If you feel bloated or distended and your waist has grown in size, this may merely represent dietary indiscretion and inadequate exercise. But it should be noted that of women who have ovarian tumors, the sudden distension of the abdomen may be the first or only warning. So, if you do exercise, the symptom of stomach distension should be promptly reviewed with your physician for a pelvic examination. And if you do not exercise, you can expect a gradual but increasing loss of abdominal wall tone. Healthy abdominal muscles form bands of tissue which support the internal organs of the body. The use of a girdle, instead of maintenance of proper muscle tone, generally provides an unhealthy substitute for exercise. Wearing a girdle will actually promote the development of a lazy musculature and lead to an increase of abdominal bulging. If you have poor abdominal muscle tone, you should take steps to correct the problem. Regular exercise offers many dividends, not the least of which is a better self-image. Good muscle tone makes for attractiveness. You are never too old to begin improving your abdominal muscle tone. But do so under supervision and guidance that will reflect your own rate of exercise tolerance. Inconsistent or zealous exercising is not beneficial and may actually be harmful.

Urinary-tract problems

Changes in the condition of a woman's urethra and bladder are common (see Figure 3).[1] The urinary tract is composed chiefly of epithelial cells, smooth muscle, and blood vessels. Epithelial cells are the "lining cells" of the body and are found on all internal and external surfaces, including the lining of the urinary tract. With declines in estrogen the epithelial lining tends to deteriorate and the muscle tone tends to diminish.[1] These changes may lead to some loss of bladder control (urinary incontinence). This may be why some menopausal women are awakened at night with an urge to urinate to a degree that they had not experienced before. Many women report the problem and find it annoying.

Not all urinary problems that women experience are of menopausal origin. Reports also suggest that some hardening of the arteries may be responsible. When this occurs, the central nervous system undergoes some deterioration, which may lead to an increased urgency to urinate during the night.[1] Whatever the cause, the loss of control of urinary function can be very distressing. Severe problems are rare and tend not to be menopausally related since the condition occurs as often in younger as in older women.[7]

Stress incontinence, the loss of urine when under stress, is relatively more common. Mild stress incontinence involves the loss of a little urine when laughing or coughing or emotionally overwrought. It is quite common among all women and seems to increase slightly with the passing years.

An exercise regimen, developed in the 1950s by Dr. A. M. Kegel, has been reported to be effective in restoring bladder control. The exercise regimen requires three twenty-minute sessions a day and consists of training a woman to tense the pubococ-

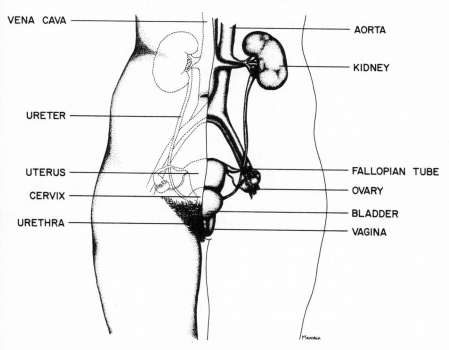

VENA CAVA

AORTA

KIDNEY

URETER

UTERUS

FALLOPIAN TUBE

CERVIX

OVARY

URETHRA

BLADDER

VAGINA

Figure 3 The Genitourinary System of Woman

cygeus muscles. These muscles form several sheets of contractile tissue in the regions around the vaginal, urethra, and anal structures. Among Dr. Kegel's first 500 cases reported, 75 percent who completed an eight-week exercise program found complete relief.[7] He noted that some of the most gratifying results were achieved among women in their eighties as well as those who had previously failed to respond to surgery.

If you are having problems with stress incontinence, you could go to a health-care professional who could place a transducer (pressure gauge) in your vagina and provide you with instructions to contract the vaginal muscles which surround the transducer. Your physician will probably find that your muscular function is less than adequate.[7] The fact is, however, that you don't need such a clinical process. *You* can locate and retrain these muscles in the privacy of your own home.

First you have to locate the pubococcygeus muscles. These are the ones that surround the vagina and anus. If you were to insert a tampon and contract the vaginal muscle (squeeze) around it, you would have located this sheet of muscle. Alternatively, contracting the anal sphincter as one would to prevent a bowel movement, will produce the tightening of these muscles. Don't worry if the first contractions seem very puny and weak. With practice, the muscles will get much stronger. Once you have found your pubococcygeus muscles, begin a practice program. One approach is to contract these muscles twenty-five to thirty times, several different times each day. Keep at it and the strength of the contractions will increase.[7] You can do the exercises throughout the day whenever you remember since no one but you need be aware that you are working on toning these muscles. The effort does not show. As the strength of the muscles increases, you will gain conscious control of the necessary muscles for bladder control. In addition, the overall muscle tone of your internal pelvic area will improve greatly. Exercise will improve your pelvic supports. More extensive vaginal relaxations often occur because of childbirth-related tissue plane weaknesses from tears and may require surgical correction if the exercises are not helpful. The simpler approach is always preferable to surgical correction. Persist in your exercise. Nonetheless, being wet from urinary loss is most unpleasant. However, before submitting to surgical correction, careful review for the specific cause of the urinary leakage is essential.[1] Moreover, you should select carefully a gynecologist with special expertise in this subspecialty of surgical gynecology.

Vaginal and reproductive gland changes

When estrogen levels drop, one of the last symptoms to appear can be vaginal regression. To test for this the physician may take a swab of fluid from the vagina and smear it onto a glass slide, thereby obtaining a "vaginal smear." Estrogenized vaginal smears look different under the microscope than atrophic (regressed) smears. These estrogenized vaginal smears do continue to occur for some women well past menopause,[20] and it is clear that not all women lose estrogen stimulation of the vaginal tissue with increasing age. Moreover, contrary to what was formerly assumed, the vaginal skin may not always be a reliable indicator of your overall estrogen blood levels. If vaginal dryness and pain on intercourse do occur, estrogen creams will be highly effective. Figure 4 shows the relationships among the ovary, tubes, uterus, and vagina.

The ovaries

As your ovaries get older, two distinct structural changes occur: they get smaller, and their composition changes. While the menopausal ovary no longer ovulates an egg each month nor continues the cycle of follicular development, ovulation, corpus-luteum development, and regression,[2] it does perform some very vital functions.[8, 9, 14, 15] The idea that an old ovary is useless is

FALLOPIAN TUBE

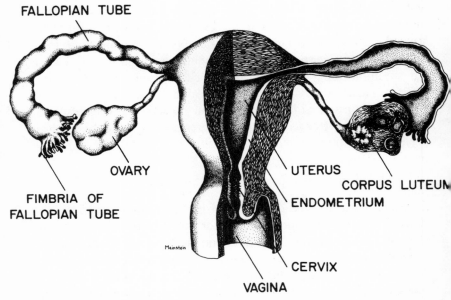

OVARY

FIMBRIA OF
FALLOPIAN TUBE

UTERUS

CORPUS LUTEUM

ENDOMETRIUM

CERVIX

VAGINA

Figure 4   The Reproductive Organs of Woman (Ovaries, Tubes, Uterus, Cervix, and Vagina)

incorrect. The cells of the older ovary look different. Look at Plates A through E (pages 41, 45, 46, 50, 51) to see how different they are.

The nonovulating ovary actively participates in the secretion of hormones: chiefly androstenedione.[12] The cortex (outer shell) of the ovary becomes thinner and wrinkled as the entire ovary is shrinking in size.[2] This is to be expected since the cortex is the region which contains the primitive cells which give rise to eggs, and by menopause the original lifetime supply of eggs is almost completely exhausted. The inner part of the ovary (stroma) is quite different. For many women these cells can be very active cells that are secreting androgen hormones: androstenedione and testosterone.[2, 4] Older ovaries often produce abundant testosterone.[10, 12, 13] Your ovaries are an important source of the hormones which promote well-being.[5] With age, the adrenal glands appear to produce estrogen in place of the ovary, but at much reduced levels.

The uterus

Your uterus, or womb, is a smooth muscle with a glandular inner surface known as the endometrium. This glandular area, in a younger cycling woman, changes monthly—building up and breaking down with each menstrual cycle. The uterus also appears to produce hormones called prostaglandins, which seem to have many influences throughout the body. Prostaglandins are produced in many body tissues. Not all of the prostaglandins' functions are completely understood.

In about half of menopausal women the endometrium begins to regress and become what is known as "senile endometrium."[16] Although all women maintain an endometrium, in some it may be more atrophic than in others depending on their own estrogen levels.

The tip of the womb, called the cervix, resides in the top of the vagina. In surveys of young women at the University of Pennsylvania as well as of perimenopausal women at Stanford University, 30 percent to 50 percent had a definite preference for deep penile thrusting during coitus. It seems, from the women's comments on the questionnaires, that they were aware of and liked direct cervical stimulation. We do know that there are sensitive nerves located in the human cervix which are the type that fire impulses to the brain after they are stimulated.[19] As the cervix ages, these nerves gradually disappear. The whole issue of uterine involvement in sexual arousal needs to be examined in light of these and three other recent reports.[3, 17, 21] Your uterus is an important part of your body. It is very likely that future research will teach us how important an organ it is—even after the childbearing years are completed.

The Fallopian tubes

At the top of your uterus, as an extension of it on either side, rise the Fallopian tubes. During the reproductive years these tubes are very vibrant, active, and dynamic organs. Each tube connects the central core of the womb to the area of the abdominal cavity which is near one of your ovaries. It is this tube which not only picks up the egg through its fingerlike ends but also it is through this tube, that the sperm swim (through the vagina, cervix, womb, and tubes) toward their rendezvous with a waiting egg to start a new life.

At menopause, when estrogen levels decline, the cellular structure of the tubes begin to regress similarly to the regression process in the uterus.[6, 18]

Summary

There are major changes in skin, urinary tract, breast, vagina, and uterus that all begin as the ovarian changes of reduced estrogens and progesterone trigger the menopausal years. The most critical changes, however, occur in your bones, and these are dealt with separately in the next chapter.

4 / The Bones and How They Grow

While the strong stuff we call bone may look solid, it is actually composed of countless numbers of molecules that are bound to each other in an ever-changing array of spongy looking but firm inner matrix and an outer compact, thinner, smooth surface. Blood vessels and nerves travel through the bone tissue just as they do through every other part of the body. Bone is comprised of calcium as well as other structural elements. Each day calcium leaves bone and enters the blood. Other molecules of calcium, traveling in the blood, are taken up into bone and add to its mass. This process forms a continuing cycle of bone remodeling (breaking down and building up), and the different phases of the remodeling cycle are controlled by a variety of hormones, including estrogen. Although most of us tend to think of our bones as structurally sound tissue that does not change, actually our bones are vital tissue whose parts are constantly breaking down and building up. To maximize healthy bone, you need an adequate daily supply of calcium.

Figure 5 illustrates how the blood vessels and nerves insert into bone. Figure 6 shows the three kinds of bone that make up the human skeleton: the long bones (for example, arms), the short bones (vertebrae from the spinal column), and the sesamoid (kneecaps).

Muscles also need calcium. If there is not enough calcium in your blood to supply your muscles adequately, your bones will give up as much of their calcium as the muscles need. The bones do this even at the expense of their own strength and health. Moreover, a certain amount of calcium is excreted in urine and feces every day, and this loss must be made up in the diet.[23, 37] It is, therefore, very important for you to consume calcium on a daily basis.

Your need for calcium

A variety of studies have shown that when you reach your menopausal years, your need for calcium is likely to increase. The reason is complex. Less of the dietary calcium gets absorbed into the body from the digestive tract as people get older.[12, 26, 19] Young people who eat less than the optimal amounts of calcium-rich foods appear to have a "fail-safe system" for increasing the calcium absorption of the foods they do ingest. Vitamin D (specifically the form called $1,25,OH_2D$) comes to the rescue by—so to speak—extracting the calcium passing through the intestines. The vitamin D increases the rate of transfer (uptake) of the calcium from the intestines into the body. Once the calcium gets across the walls of the intestines, it enters the blood stream and travels through the body like hormones do when traveling in blood. When people get older, this fail-safe backup system becomes less efficient. It, therefore, is critically important that the diet supply enough calcium for the needs of the body when people are older.

If you are menopausal, the RDA (recommended daily allowance) for calcium that is listed by the Food and Drug Administra-

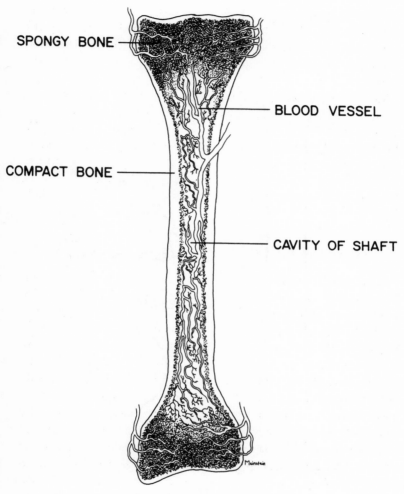

Figure 5 Bone Structure

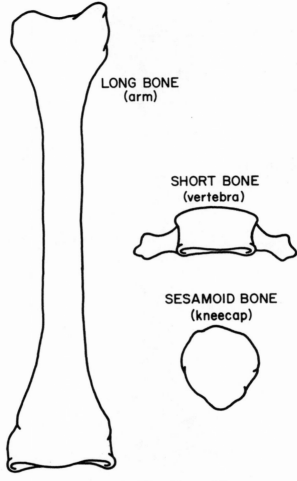

LONG BONE
(arm)

SHORT BONE
(vertebra)

SESAMOID BONE
(kneecap)

Figure 6 The Three Types of Bone

tion is probably too low for you. Ignore the nutritional charts on the food packages you buy. They are given in percentages rather than in milligrams (mg.), and the percentages may be based on the RDA of 600 mg. per day—too low for a menopausal woman.

Exactly how much calcium you need will vary according to your unique metabolic requirements. To be safe, you should ingest about 1,000 mg. a day in order to prevent a loss of bone mass due to dietary inadequacy.[14, 37] But do not overdo it. Be sure to stay within a conservative range because excessive calcium could create other problems. People who have excessive blood levels of calcium show a tendency to calcification of arterial areas (promoting arteriosclerosis) and kidney stones. Moderation is the key. You can supply your calcium in an orderly fashion by looking at Appendix 3 to find which calcium-rich foods you prefer. The calorie content of each is also listed to help you plan. Three glasses of skim milk a day will suffice; or any other combination that provides the total needed.

Unfortunately most women do not consume enough of this essential mineral. Large-scale studies have shown that women, on average, consume less than half of the calcium that they need.[3] One reason that some women don't drink enough milk to satisfy calcium requirements is that excessive milk drinking seems to upset their stomach.[6] Skim milk might be better digested. It will be as valuable to your bone. But if you feel this way about all forms of milk, check Appendix 3 for other sources of calcium that you might digest more comfortably. If you find nothing that suits you, you should take calcium in tablet form. Calcium can be purchased without prescription. Several different brands are available, and some combine calcium and protein within one pill.

How menopause affects your bones

As we have previously explained, at menopause your estrogen levels are likely to start a long and continuous decline. Since each woman is different, not every woman will have the loss. But the vast majority will. We now know that it is a combination of estrogen and calcium deficiencies that together accelerate bone deterioration.

Osteoporosis

Whenever estrogen levels fall drastically, whether due to natural menopause or surgical removal of the estrogen supply (ovariectomy), bones begin losing mass.[33] A number of reports have shown this loss of mass to vary from about .5 percent to 3 percent per year.[16, 37] The bones become progressively thinner in the vast majority of menopausal women not taking replacement estrogen.[20] By the time a woman is eighty, she can easily have lost 40 percent of her bone substance.[34, 36] Although men also suffer some loss, theirs is not as devastating as that of women.[34] While their loss of bone mass is as great, breaks occur much less often apparently because men start out with larger bones. For women the greatest declines in bone mass occur between the ages of forty-five and seventy. By age sixty at least half of all women, in every country now studied, show osteoporosis when X-rayed.[20]

Estrogen plays an important role in bone metabolism. Remember that bone is always exchanging calcium with the blood. Two ways estrogen influences this exchange process are (1) by facilitating the uptake of calcium from the blood into the bone and (2) by inhibiting the loss of calcium from bone. When estrogen levels fall, the bones begin to disintegrate. *Osteoporosis* means "increased porosity." Think of the "pores" in Swiss cheese and imagine them enlarging, and you will have a reasonable analogy to bone porosity. Osteoporosis is the disease characterized by a decrease in mass so great that as the porosity increases, fractures begin to occur even without severe trauma or concussion. For a woman with osteoporosis of the spine, a gentle hug can break her spinal bones.

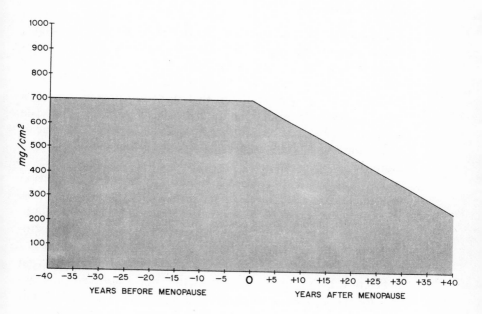

Figure 7 Declines in Bone Mass Begin at Menopause—and Continue
From Meema *et al., Obstet and Gynecol* 26:333.

Spinal fractures

Take a look at Figure 7. It shows that once menopause begins, loss of bone ensues and this loss continues as long as the estrogen levels remain below bone maintenance requirements.[4, 32, 33, 36]

Figures 8 and 9 show the effect of age on the density of bone for men and for women. Note that in young people there is a trend toward increasing bone mass each year with age. The scale (inches $\times$ 10^{-3}) is very technical and not relevant to the issue of increasing and subsequent decreasing of bone mass with age. (For more detail, see reference 7.)

The problem of bone loss is not simply or inevitably a condition of aging. Most of the studies have shown that when women take estrogens, they do not lose bone mass, provided they continue to take the hormones.[33, 37] But for women who do not take estrogen, bone loss commonly occurs; and when it does, the degree of the loss of bone occurs in proportion to the degree of the estrogen deficiency. Deterioration of bone is the single most critical problem for menopausal women. In fact, it has been estimated that about 50 percent of all women will develop some degree of osteoporosis after menopause.

The earliest warning symptom is a backache in the lower part of the spine—a progressive and persistent pain that seldom radiates.[3] Most aches and pains tend to spread (radiate). If you notice a constant, localized pain in your lower back, take the pain as a warning sign and seek treatment from an orthopedic specialist or knowledgeable gynecologist.[5] On average, those who do develop the disease begin to notice more severe backaches about 9½ years after their last menstrual period or 13 years after a surgically induced menopause.[8] The spine and pelvic bones are generally, but not always, affected first.[8]

Spinal osteoporosis is rarely diagnosed before spinal bones have broken. The breaks follow a very orderly pattern, which leads to the appearance of the so-called "Dowager's Hump."[43] The Dow-

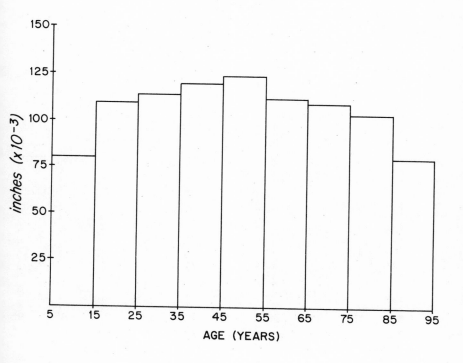

Figure 8 Changes in Bone Density with Age: Men
From Albanese *et al., NY State J Med* (1975):326–336.

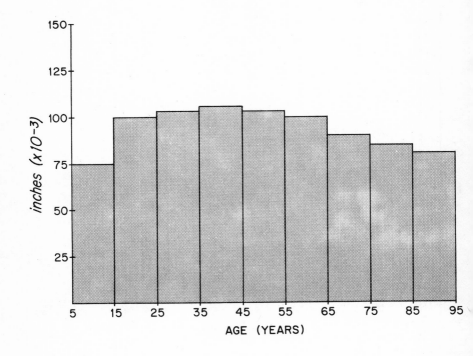

Figure 9   Changes in Bone Density with Age: Women
From Albanese *et al.*, NY State J Med (1975):326–336.

ager's Hump, that protrusion in the upper back that can give an older woman the appearance of being a hunchback, is one of the clear indications of osteoporosis.[2] On average, at around age sixty, then again at sixty-five and seventy, an afflicted woman suffers breaks. The breaks occur at the places where the spine naturally curves (see Figure 10). These are the weakest points in one's spinal column, and these are the first to break. After the bones break the body forms a fat pad over the spine in the region of the fractures to compensate, and this adds to the deformity. Figure 11 illustrates the resulting change in posture and height that follow the breakage shown in Figure 10.

Hip fractures

Hip fractures due to osteoporosis occur in 30 percent of all women after age sixty-five. Figure 12 shows the long hip bone—the femur. Note that the top region—the hip socket—has a notched area where the hip bones rest. This notched area is the weakest part of this large bone because it is the thinnest, and it receives the stress of supporting the upper part of the body. When bones become porous and fragile, this spot is vulnerable to fracture. If the bone is thin enough, the mildest bump can break it. As of 1974, 10 percent to 15 percent of those women who suffered a hip fracture died within four months of the fracture.[22, 9] Although the causes of death vary, the lion's share includes four: viral pneumonia, myocardial infarction, cerebro-vascular accident, and heart failure.[10a] There has been a great improvement in surgical correction of bone fracture in the last eight to ten years and this 15 percent death rate may no longer be correct. New studies have not yet evaluated whether the prognosis has improved. But even for those who don't die, the consequences of hip fracture are extremely serious. Life as a cripple in a wheel chair, loss of independence, loss of freedom of movement and travel, all combine to make this a terrible disease indeed.

Hip fractures occur more often in some geographical regions

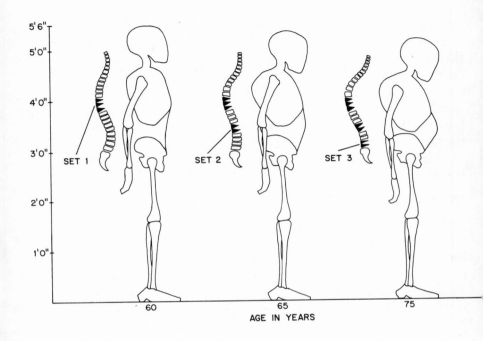

Figure 10 Spinal Osteoporosis—Location of Bone Fracture with Resulting Postural Changes
From Urist, *Clinics Endocrinol Metab* 2:159–176.

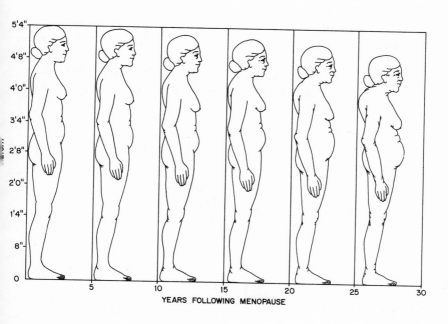

YEARS FOLLOWING MENOPAUSE

Figure 11 Postural Changes Associated with Spinal Osteoporosis and the Dowager's Hump
From A. Albanese, *Postgraduate Medicine* 63:167–172.

than in others. Women in Scandinavia and England show much higher rates than those in China or South Africa.[13] Whether this variation is due to differences in sunlight (which increases vitamin-D production on one's skin), to physical activity patterns (which promote better muscle tone, thereby supporting and protecting fragile bones), or to hormonal variation among differ-

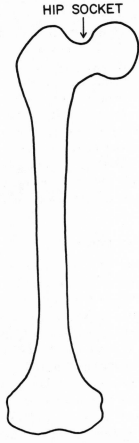

HIP SOCKET

Figure 12   The Femur

ent races has not yet been resolved. Most likely all three factors contribute.

Loss of teeth

Other effects of a loss of bone mass are found in the mouth. Your teeth are supported by bone, and, not surprisingly, periodontal disease (the loss of tooth-bearing bone) is quite common in osteoporotic women.[7] In fact, by age sixty about 40 percent of women will have lost all their teeth, according to one investigator who studied thousands of otherwise healthy women.[6] Whether this dental problem is due solely to osteoporosis or to some interaction with poor dental hygiene is not yet resolved. But daily gum care through flossing and/or use of a water pick is an essential part of fastidious grooming. If you have not been incorporating daily removal of debris from the base of your gums before, it becomes critical that you do so now. A toothbrush cannot retrieve food particles that work their way down below the gum line, and these particles provide the nutrition source for odorous bacteria that will grow in the mouth if the food remains more than twenty-four hours at a time.

Osteoporosis becomes obvious

The usual precipitating symptom of osteoporosis that brings a woman to the attention of her doctor is a bone that breaks after a minor jolt. The broken bone causes pain. The woman seeks medical help. And an X-ray shows the overall deterioration of her bones.[8] The bones break easily because, through the gradual loss of mass, they have become brittle. Women whose ovaries are removed (regardless of the age) begin to show osteoporosis within two years after the operation if no hormone replacement therapy is instituted.[25] Studies conducted four years after the operation showed that 68 percent of one group of 59 ovariectomized women were suffering from beginning osteoporosis.

Since the loss of estrogen following ovariectomy carries with it an increased risk of osteoporosis, it is not very surprising that the estrogen decline of menopause is also likely to lead to the development of osteoporosis. But even after menopause, there is wide variation in blood hormone levels among women. Two studies compared hormone levels of postmenopausal women, some of whom had the disease and some of whom did not have it. Clear differences emerged. Although estradiol and testosterone levels were not different in the two groups, levels of estrone and androstenedione were significantly lower in the women with osteoporosis.[17, 31] In other words, menopausal women with relatively high levels of androstenedione and estrone are less likely to suffer the ravaging effects of osteoporosis. Estrone, therefore, appears to be the estrogen hormone by which bone health can be maintained in menopause. Recall that the menopausal ovary secretes both estrone and androstenedione. Some women produce more than others. In some menopausal women, the ovaries are probably quite important in preventing or delaying the onset of osteoporosis. Here is another good reason to keep your ovaries intact even if a hysterectomy (removal of the uterus) becomes advisable.

How the disease is diagnosed

If you suspect that your bones are disintegrating (because your height is shrinking or your back is causing persistent pain), you can go to a physician for a bone reading. Many different methods are available to check your bone density. Most are painless and quick and involve a form of X-ray visualization of some of your bone. A bone densitometer is a small machine about the size of a typewriter. The technician will guide your arm through a cuff, much as in blood-pressure recording. A small beam of photons that you can't see or feel is passed through your arm, and a minicomputer, attached to the machine, calculates how dense your bone is. If you do have the disease, it will be occurring in a number of places simultaneously rather than in just one location. The fingers, spine, lower arm, and hip bones are all affected once osteoporosis is well progressed, and accurate readings can be taken from any of these regions.

Menopausal risk factors

If you are childless, white, small-boned, and slender your risk of developing the disease is much greater than if you have had children, are black, or large-boned, or chubby.[3, 8, 9, 34] There is an enormous individual variation in the ability of the body to maintain its bone density, and about half of menopausal women do not experience any ill effects of menopause on their bones.[36] Even for those in the high-risk categories, estrogens appear to prevent osteoporosis as long as the hormone treatment continues.

Treatments for osteoporosis

As in any disease, the best treatment is prevention. Those who maintain adequate exercise and nutrition will have the least risk of getting osteoporosis. Moreover, hormone therapy will almost always prevent the disease, provided the calcium levels are adequate. Once the disease has been diagnosed, treatment will, optimally, consist of vitamin D, adequate calcium intake (at least 1,000 mg. per day), and some estrogen supplements. Current scientific research is evaluating other approaches such as calcitonin injections and sodium-fluoride treatments. Ultimately, the goal of bone treatment involves controlling the delicate balance between bone formation and bone resorption (breakdown).

Some controversy exists about the nature of treatment. While almost all experts agree that estrogen is effective, investigations are under way to determine if other agents will also work. Fluoride treatment, for example, appeared effective. When coupled with estrogen fluoride promotes bone growth.[41] However, it seems that the new bone that is formed with fluoride treatment has been reported to break easily.[14, 40] About 40 percent of the women taking the fluoride developed severe enough side effects (rheumatic pains, nausea, and vomiting) to stop treatment.[41] We suggest that you avoid sodium-fluoride treatments at this time. Some investigators believe that estrogen is the treatment of choice, with or without calcitonin (another bone-related hormone) supplements.[15] Calcitonin is one of the lesser-known hormones of the thyroid gland and is important in the control of bone function.[38] This therapy is new; treatment with calcitonin requires frequent injections, and one of the serious objections to this treatment involves antibody reactions which have not yet been worked out.[14, 15] The calcitonin that is injected into the women comes from a nonhuman source and is viewed as a foreign invasion by the women's white blood cells; the body response, in this case, is to manufacture antibodies which attack the injected calcitonin. In time, calcitonin may come to be beneficial for treatment of osteoporosis in menopausal women. Right now it is experimental. Estrogen therapy increases a woman's natural levels of calcitonin.

There are a few investigators who believe that estrogens are irrelevant but that calcium and vitamin-D therapy are sufficient to protect against or even reverse the disease.[7] Theirs is the weakest case to support with hard evidence. Still others have been advocating calcitonin and phosphate (a naturally occurring substance) combination therapy. The sensible approach in our opinion, after giving full consideration to the available evidence, appears to be one that assures *adequate exercise* as well as adequate calcium levels (1,000 mg. per day), sufficient vitamin D (400 IU per day) or fifteen minutes of unpolluted sun shining on your skin), and enough estrogen to maintain the retention of bone mass. If you live in an area of great air pollution, sunning yourself may not give you the necessary wave lengths of solar radiation to reach your skin. If in doubt, a vitamin source or milk (which in the United States contains D supplements) provides assurance of adequate ingestion.

Estrogen therapy is particularly important because it reduces the net loss of calcium from the body.[21] In fact, calcium loss can be cut by even very low doses of estrogens. Doses of estrogen that are too high cause the body to retain too much calcium. As described earlier, excess calcium may create other problems with the kidneys (stones) or the circulatory system (calcium deposits clogging the arteries). Again, with estrogen, moderation is the key.

It has been demonstrated in a number of studies that estrogen therapy helps bone to maintain its mineral strength and mass. Among normal, healthy, menopausal women tested for up to eight years, the estrogen-treated women still had as much bone as they had started with years earlier, but the placebo-treated women has lost as much as 9 percent of their bone after eight years.[18, 29, 33]

Estrogens work better than placebo and better than calcium alone. This is graphically illustrated in Figure 13. Note how each treatment is associated with some decline of bone (reflected in the loss of height) as the years pass, but that some treatments have much less decline than other treatments.

In other controlled studies in which women were given placebos, hormones, or calcium, clear differences emerged after two years. The control subjects taking a placebo lost an average of 1.18 percent to 2.83 percent of their bone mass per year (depending on which of two measuring techniques was considered). Calcium (calcium carbonate) was effective in reducing bone loss to about one-fifth that of untreated women. However the estrogen treatment was the single most effective agent. It reduced bone loss to half that of the calcium-treated group.[14, 16, 24] Estrogen therapy in low doses (.3 or .6 mg. per day) does not produce side effects for the vast majority of women. If side effects occur (like a bloated feeling or swollen breasts), this usually indicates that the dose of estrogen is too high. Adjustments are made immediately, either

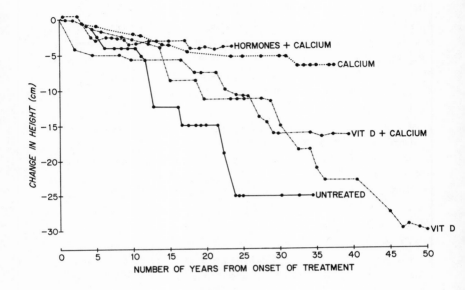

Figure 13   Changes in Height of Menopausal Women in Response to Different Treatments
From Nordin *et al.*, *Clin Orthop and Rel Res* 140:216–239.

by alternating days of therapy (a day on, a day off) or by halving the daily dose.

You're likely to find that your choice of a physician will define which treatment you are offered. The medical community has not reached a consensus on how best to treat or prevent the condition. By mid-1981, a questionnaire reply by 1,000 specialists showed that only 42 percent used hormone therapy even for treatment of diagnosed osteoporosis.[11] Vitamin D was prescribed by half of those who advocate estrogen treatment for osteoporosis.

By becoming informed, you can increase the scope of your own health care. Here are the suggestions:

1. Develop and maintain good exercise habits. Exercise habits appear to play a role in preventing the disease. In countries where women are engaged in physical work up to an advanced age, the incidence of age-related bone fractures is significantly reduced.[10] The reverse situation, immobilization, has been related to a high incidence of the disease.[7]

While there is a general impression in the biomedical community that the more active you are, the stronger your bones will be, the actual studies make a subtly different point. Total immobility (hospitalized bed rest) does produce loss of bone mass.[7, 23] In the opposite condition, extreme activity in a particular limb—as, for example, in the throwing arm of a baseball player—increased bone mass in the heavily used limb occurs.[44] But the two studies which compared the bone mass of active menopausal women to the bone mass of less active individuals failed to find the expected difference.[20, 42] So while extremes of activity do relate to bone mass, varying amounts of activity, within the normal range found among a large sample of menopausal women, do not necessarily change bone mass. However, regular exercise will promote greater muscle tone and mass. This increased muscle will serve to cushion and support the bones and will be an especially important benefit to women whose bone mass is declining.

2. Maintain an adequate daily intake of calcium—1,000 mg. per day should be enough. This can be achieved by consuming three glasses of milk or three ounces of Swiss cheese per day or by other means. If your calcium intake is deficient, increasing your intake will stop (and possibly reverse) the loss of bone mass.[2, 67, 11, 28] Appendix 3 lists the calcium value of the common best food sources.

3. Be sure you have a moderate supply of vitamin D. Too little or too much is bad—but for different reasons. In moderate amounts vitamin D promotes the uptake of the calcium you have eaten from the intestines into the blood stream. If your vitamin-D level is too low, the calcium you ingest won't be absorbed into the body. Instead, it is likely to be lost in the feces.[14] You can maintain an adequate intake of vitamin D by either exposing your skin for about fifteen minutes a day to the sun or by drinking milk (to which vitamin D has been added) or by taking a vitamin pill. Again, moderation is the key. Fifteen minutes of sun exposure with no sunscreen on your skin to block the rays[1] is good in that your skin will manufacture the necessary vitamin D. Excessive sun exposure is destructive to the skin, burning away the melanocyte cells that protect you. Moreover, in amounts above 1,000 IU per day, vitamin D promotes an excess release of calcium from bone into the blood.[14, 39] This causes a loss of bone mass. The appropriate amount is 400 IU of vitamin D per day.

The ability of vitamin D to halt or reverse an osteoporotic condition is limited by the level of estrogen deficiency that is present.[11] If you have too little estrogen in your system, vitamin D won't help. It sounds more complicated than it really is. You need calcium for your bone mass. You need vitamin D to help get the calcium into the body but not so much that the calcium stays in the blood rather than the bone. You need estrogen to keep the calcium inside the bones. Shortages in any of these requirements or excesses in vitamin D can cause your bones to become brittle.

4. Be aware of your height. If you start to shrink, you are probably losing bone. If you are maintaining adequate amounts of calcium, additional estrogen supplements will help. You don't need a lot of estrogen to do the job of keeping your bones intact. The lowest doses (.3 mg. per day) on the market will be adequate. See Table 1 on pages 114–115 for a list of kinds and dosages of estrogen. Any brand's lowest dose will provide as much as you need for your bones.

5. Consider estrogen therapy as prevention if there is a risk of bone deterioration, but be sure that your calcium levels are also adequate.

How much estrogen is appropriate?

Since there is great individual variation in the amount of circulating estrone different menopausal women show, there is no "proper" dose of estrogen that should be universally prescribed to correct or prevent osteoporosis. Even the lowest doses usually prescribed (.3 mg. per day of conjugated estrogen) have been shown to be adequate.[21] So far all of the estrogen studies have used oral estrogens, so the effectiveness of other forms (tablets placed under the tongue and vaginal creams) remains untested. However, since blood levels of estrone appear to be a critical predictor of bone health, and all forms of estrogen treatment lead to significant increases in blood levels of estrone, it is likely that estrogen therapy in any form will be beneficial for bone health.

Your doctor may suggest that you take progesterone if hormone therapy seems advisable and your uterus has not been removed. Although progesterone is important in preventing adverse effects of estrogen (see Chapter 6), it will not prevent bone loss that is caused by an estrogen deficiency.[18, 30] Androgen is different. It seems to be about as effective as estrogen in halting bone deterioration,[14, 27] but the possibility of masculinizing (for example, causing growth of facial hair) makes this a less desirable hormone treatment than estrogen.

Hormone therapy is generally necessary to halt and reverse the degenerative process of the disease in the presence of adequate levels of vitamin-D intake. A variety of studies confirm this.[14, 16, 29, 35] For example, in one group of thirty women who were beginning to show annual loss of their bone mass, those subjects given a placebo showed about 3.6 percent degeneration of their (finger) bones each year. In contrast, the groups given either estrogen therapy or estrogen plus progesterone showed no bone loss, and some of the women actually showed a slightly increased bone density at the end of the first year.[30] Another report indicated that women who began taking estrogens within three years after their last menstrual period and who continued taking them for ten years thereafter showed a slight increase in bone mass after the ten years had passed. Those who began estrogens later, after having advanced more than three years into their menopause, stopped losing bone but were not able to regain any of the bone mass lost.[35] Different studies have reported different annual rates, but all show a clear tendency for bone loss which is progressive when no hormones are taken.

Summary

Osteoporosis is the most dangerous malady of the menopausal years. Bones become progressively thinner and more brittle and are subject to fractures as menopause progresses. The relative paucity of estrogen during the menopausal years appears to play a major role in the development of this devastating disease. Calcium inadequacies and lack of exercise are also critical factors. Hormone therapy with estrogen can prevent the occurrence of osteoporosis and even retard the condition once it has started. There is growing evidence that those who begin taking estrogen early in their menopausal years may even show a slight increase in their bone mass over time. If you do take estrogen, you will need to take it as long as you want to prevent further bone loss. As far as your bone health is concerned, the findings are unambiguous. If you are at risk of bone deterioration, estrogen therapy provides a clear benefit.

5 / Hormone Replacement Therapy I

Hormone replacement therapy. The words seem to suggest that menopause is a condition of loss. And for most women this is true. Hormone levels decline as the ovaries shrink with age; and as they shrink, the menopausal symptoms discussed earlier begin to appear. But the hot flashes and night sweats are only the tip of the iceberg. They really herald an underlying estrogen deficiency that, if unchecked, is likely to set in motion the bone-degeneration processes and other body changes that were described in the previous chapters.

Said one woman of sixty:

I approached menopause with a firm determination that this was not going to affect my life! I was sadly disillusioned! I found that the hot flashes did bother me and I was reduced to the emotional level of a young teenager—the least little thing bothered me. I sought the advice of a gynecologist who put me on Premarin [a conjugated estrogen]. That was

10 years ago and I have been fine ever since—feeling good emotionally and physically.

    Having a large percentage of menopausal women is natural for a society in which the average life span is seventy years or more. When antibiotics were developed to kill man's killers, no one said that it was unnatural to promote well-being by killing disease. The drugs ended a common form of death (by infection) that had prevented women from reaching their menopause. As health conditions improved over the last two centuries, few thought it unnatural to improve conditions that lead to longevity. No one suggested that heat and shelter, packaged food and medicine were unnatural. These things increased longevity, and with longevity came menopause.

    The development of estrogen therapy is a recent biomedical innovation. The modern study of hormones—how they work, where they are produced, what their benefits are—began in the 1940s. It has brought us the understanding that hormones are natural body secretions that control many of the physiological processes of life. Hormone replacement therapy (HRT) for menopausal symptoms has been praised as well as maligned. Like any other tool of medicine and science, used correctly in the appropriate circumstances its effects are beneficial. The issues involved in HRT are:

- Does HRT relieve the symptoms of menopausal distress?
- What are the side effects of HRT?
- How does one take HRT?
- What constitutes a beneficial dosage of hormones?
- What route of administration is best (oral pills, vaginal creams, or sublingual tablets)?
- What about progesterone?

- What kinds of dosages of estrogen are available?
- Who should not use HRT? (See Chapter 6.)

HRT and relief from menopausal distress

Too little estrogen appears to be the principal cause of hot flashes, usually the first symptom of menopausal distress. Estrogen treatment almost always relieves them. The studies are absolutely unambiguous on this point. If you have no symptoms, your hormone levels are probably adequate to maintain the health of your bones as well as your general well being. You are very fortunate. Women who do have hot flashes, tingling, genital atrophy, or night sweats find relief when they take estrogen, regardless of the form in which it is taken.

Hot flashes

The proof that hormone therapy is far superior to placebo, sedatives, or clonidine (an antihypertensive drug) in relieving hot flashes and night sweats is contained in Appendix 1. For a full discussion please turn there.

Some women take vitamin E in the belief that it helps to relieve hot flashes. But according to rigorous scientific studies, it just does not work.[23] Likewise, others believe that a woman who exercises regularly may be less prone to hot flashes. Exercise, although good for you in other ways, does not help to alleviate the hot flashes.[9] With time, even without hormones hot flashes do diminish, although many women continue to experience flashing for ten years or more.

Genital skin atrophy

If you are suffering from hormonal deficits that produce vaginal dryness or painful intercourse, taking estrogen will probably solve the problem entirely.[17, 18] The pressure of a thrusting penis in an inadequately lubricated vagina with a thin epithelial lining can produce abrasions. Abrasions of the vaginal lining lead to inflammation, and this inflammation is commonly seen in women who have estrogen deficiencies. But you will have to continue taking the estrogen to maintain relief. If you stop, your estrogen level will drop and the problems will probably return. Estrogen can be prescribed in different forms (vaginal cream, oral pill, under-the-tongue tablet). The effectiveness of a given dose is related to the type of estrogen that is taken. One investigator treated forty-two women with atrophic vaginitis (vaginal inflammation with inadequate secretions and a general wasting-away appearance). The study was rigorously carried out in double-blind fashion: neither the patients nor the person evaluating results knew until the study ended who got the hormone and who got the blank (placebo) treatment. A daily dose of .1 mg. of estradiol (the most active form of estrogen) in cream form was sufficient to maintain vaginal normalcy.[18] The necessary dose in pill form probably varies in different women. In two studies 1.25 mg. (conjugated equine estrogen) or more per day was needed to return the deteriorating vaginal cells to a vigorous state.[8, 17] In a more recent report (1982), .625 mg. per day provided adequate protection.[37a] In contrast to vaginal atrophy, pelvic tone is usually not restored by hormone therapy.[38] Those women who suffer from vaginal relaxation—a general loss of internal support structure strength—need other therapy. Loss of vaginal muscle tone is more common in women who have borne many children and apparently is not a reflection of hormonal deficits. Recall that the Kegel exercises (see page 75) not only help restore muscle tone but you can do them yourself.[22] You might be wise to try this before seeking medical help.

Facial skin

The skin of your face will also respond to estrogen therapy, and it, like the vaginal skin, will benefit with increased tone and glow and thickness.[21, 29, 30, 31]

Backache

Osteoporosis is a common menopausal problem that was described in Chapter 4. It affects in some way about half of the women who do not take estrogen. It is progressive (it gets worse) and is prevented by early application and continued maintenance of estrogen therapy (see Chapter 4). Backache can be an early warning sign of incipient osteoporosis—i.e., thinning out of bone.

Emotional distress

Your sense of well-being is likely to improve if you take estrogens. If you have been plagued with hot flashes and other assorted ills, obtaining some relief from them should go a long way toward making you feel a lot better. A sense of well-being is a subtly identified state. If you have it, there is an internal comfort, a ready smile, and a general feeling of good will toward oneself and others. Estrogen deficits at menopause have been shown to be associated with a loss of this comfortable feeling, and this loss is a menopausal symptom that is quite different from the other distressing symptoms. Hormone replacement therapy appears to restore this sense of well-being.[14] It also improves the quality of your sleep. In studies in sleep laboratories in England it was shown that estrogens changed the proportion of the sleep time spent in the rapid-eye-movement stage, which is characteristic of dreaming. Women dreamed more when they took estrogen and dreamed less when they were estrogen-deficient. As dreams increase, one's general state of peacefulness improves and one feels rested the next morning.[40, 41, 42] We do not yet know exactly why dream deprivation alters the psychological milieu. It may be that dreams serve to alter the electrical state of the nervous system for the better. The electrical patterns of brain waves are quite different in dream sleep than in the other stages of (nondream) sleep.

Many menopausal women report headaches, depression, anxiety, and listlessness. These symptoms are experienced by most people at one time or another and are not necessarily related to the hormone changes of the menopause. Still, this cluster of problems tends to vanish within a month or so after hormone therapy begins.[37] Placebos don't work—only the hormones do.[11] Thus, if you are suffering from a hormonal deficit and generally feeling down, hormones will work to restore your sense of vigor. But if you are having a severe emotional problem, caused by a serious life situation such as the death of a loved one or strains in your marriage, hormones probably won't help.[37]

Formication

Two years after menopause, about 10 percent of women continued to be annoyed with this itching problem for more than ten years. Estrogen treatments are the *only* remedy that reliably provides relief.[23]

Libido

Although there is a general impression within the biomedical community that HRT has some influence on libido,[2, 39] no rigorous documentation for this has yet appeared. The few reports that have been widely quoted were never explained well enough in the scientific journals to allow others to test the results by duplicating them. Until independent laboratories duplicate this work, we, as conservative professionals, listen but prefer to consider the ideas tentative.

What are the side effects of HRT?

Immediate changes for the worse in the way you feel are important to consider and deal with promptly. If you feel bad when you are taking hormones to feel good, something is wrong and you should seek an adjustment in your prescription.

Women who take estrogen don't usually experience any discomforts unless the dose is too high. If the estrogen dose is too high, there may be side effects such as breast tenderness, more vaginal discharge due to large increases in cervical secretions, weight increases, leg cramps, edema (fluid retention), headache, and unscheduled uterine bleedings.[1, 25, 42] These symptoms of overdose can continue for as long as the overdose is maintained.[24] With lower doses, side effects disappear. The overdose discomfort is entirely unnecessary. If you take estrogen and experience any of these discomforts, you should work with your doctor to determine the dosage that will make you most comfortable. Generally, there is an ideal level of hormone that is best for each individual. If it is too high, you feel overdose effects. If it is too low, you feel the menopausal distress symptoms. Your body will tell you when you are at the correct dose if you learn to listen to it.

If you take hormones for a year or more, you may need vitamin supplements. Estrogen uses up your vitamin B_6 quickly. When vitamin B_6 is depleted, depression can result. This depression is easily cured by supplementing your diet with B_6. The proper dose appears to be 100 mg. per day. If you take more than you need, the excess is excreted in the urine.[6, 19, 20, 33, 40]

One of the reasons that women live longer than men lies in their reduced incidence of heart disease before menopause. At the menopause, when estrogen levels decline, the rate of heart disease for women begins to approach the (much higher) rate for men. Although there are some data suggesting that there is an increased rate of heart disease after age forty in menstruating women on oral contraceptives (which contain hormones), the use of hormones at menopause is clearly different. With few exceptions, menopausal women who take estrogen have less heart disease, no elevation in either systolic or diastolic blood pressure, reduced cholesterol levels, and alterations of blood lipoproteins consistent with reduced risk of heart disease.

In order to avoid being an exception, you should understand the precautions. There are two of them. (1) You should have your blood pressure monitored to be certain that you are not one of the rare individuals whose blood pressure increases on estrogen (details of the studies of cardiovascular health and hormones are given in Appendix 2). (2) You should confine estrogen therapy to natural estrogen. "Natural estrogens" are those that are chemically identical to the kind that occur in nature. Some are derived from animal sources; others are made in the laboratory. In contrast, "synthetic estrogens" are those that are dissimilar to the natural ones—perhaps by as little as one atom. The distinction between natural and synthetic estrogen is relevant in the selection of a safe HRT regimen. Natural estrogens appear to be safer than synthetic estrogens. Synthetic estrogens (like ethinyl estradiol) sometimes increase the risk of cardiovascular diseases.[3, 27] Moreover, the cardiovascular benefits that accrue to estrogen only apply to the natural estrogens like Premarin, Harmogen (a brand used in Great Britain), and Estrace. For a more extensive list of which hormones are natural and which are synthetic, refer to Table 1.

Your ability to withstand infection is largely a function of how efficient your immune system is at fighting the myriad diseases to which you are constantly exposed. There is some evidence that estrogen helps stimulate immunity.[15] Experiments with guinea pigs conducted by Dr. George Feigen, a physiologist at Stanford University, explored relationships between estrogens and antibodies. Antibodies are blood-borne substances that attack infectious molecules. In guinea pigs estrogens increase the speed with which antibodies are produced and also act to lower the speed of antibody decay. This improves immunity because the antibodies remain around longer to attack infectious molecules. It seems likely that some kind of increased immune responsiveness might account for the better health in the menopausal women who take hormones. This includes lower rates of breast cancer for most groups that have been studied, as is detailed in the next chapter (immune response is relevant to cancers), and longer life spans.[7]

TABLE 1.

Kinds and Dosages of Estrogen Available:
A List of Current Products Being Sold by Prescription

We have avoided mention of brand names in this list of estrogen preparations. Throughout the text, however, we have included specific brands when referring to specific research studies that tested one or another of them. Because each may be slightly different than the other, it seems appropriate to indicate which particular form was under study.

CHEMICAL NAME	AVAILABLE PREPARATIONS
Natural estrogens	
17β-Estradiol	Tablets for oral use (doses vary by brand)
*17β-Estradiol valerate	Tablets for oral use (doses vary by brand)
Estriol	Cream, lotion, tablets (doses vary by brand)
Conjugated estrogens (equine)	Cream for vaginal application: 2.5 mg. = full applicator; 1.25 mg. = half applicator; 0.625 mg. = quarter applicator. Tablets for oral use: .3, .6, 1.25, or 2.5 mg. per pill
Estrone	Tablets for oral use: 400 mcg. to 1.5 mg. per pill
Piperazine estrone sulfate	Tablets for oral use: .625 mg. to 5 mg. per pill
Synthetic estrogens	
Ethinyl estradiol (EE)	Tablets for oral use or capsules: 10 to 50 mcg. per pill
Mestranol (not in U.S.)	Tablets for oral use or capsules (doses vary by brand)
Quinestrol	Tablets for oral use or capsules (doses vary by brand)
Diethylstilbestrol (DES)	Tablets for oral use or capsules: 200 to 500 mcg. per pill

TABLE 1 *(continued)*

CHEMICAL NAME	AVAILABLE PREPARATIONS
Chlorotrianisene (TACE)	12 to 25 mg. per pill
Clomiphene	Tablets for oral use or capsules

*Synthetic hormone in the strict sense. In the body it is converted.

Source: see references 10, 11, 13, 14, 16. Also University of Pennsylvania Hospital, Department of Pharmacology.

How does one take HRT?

In order to treat the symptoms of menopause, hormones are usually prescribed by the physician in one of three different ways. The hormones can be swallowed in pill form; taken as a wafer placed under the tongue, where it quickly melts into the skin surface, avoiding the digestive tract; or applied directly into the vagina in the form of a cream. When you take a pill, the hormone enters the blood by a different route than when you take a wafer or use a cream. The pill is swallowed, dissolves, and then passes through your stomach and out into the intestines. Once the dissolved pill is moving through the intestinal tract, normal absorption occurs, bringing the hormone across the walls of the intestine into the liver and finally into the blood stream.

The wafer, placed under the tongue (sublingual), is different. The hormone is absorbed through the cells of the mouth, moves directly into the blood stream, and only reaches the liver after it has been diluted by mixing with blood as it circulates through your blood stream.

Hormone administration by vaginal delivery is newer. The way it works is simple. You apply cream with a plunger in much the same way as you insert a menstrual tampon. The cream coats the vaginal lining and is absorbed through the walls of the vagina and moves into the blood stream. Once absorbed the estrogens appear to be diluted immediately so that no single organ except for the vagina receives a particularly high dose. Within four hours of applying the cream, the blood levels of estradiol and estrone reach the maximum levels they will attain.[32] Since standing or moving about may cause the cream to leak out of the vagina, the cream is applied at bedtime to counteract the force of gravity. When one is lying down, the hormone can be absorbed through the vaginal walls most completely.

What constitutes a beneficial dosage?

If you use hormones, you should work with your physician to find the smallest amount that is effective. For hot flashes a series of experiments[35, 36] have now defined the usual effective doses. The usual effective vaginal doses are now .2 mg. of pure estradiol or 1.25 mg. of conjugated estrogen cream (a mix of estrogen and other natural products made from the urine of pregnant mares). The pure estradiol cream comes in 1 mg. and 2 mg. applicator quantities. The dose you receive depends on whether you use a quarter, a half, or a full applicator. A .5 mg. dose of vaginal estriol (E3), the weakest of the estrogens,[36] also seems to be safe and effective. Oral doses that are effective also vary with each woman, but commonly .3 mg. or .625 mg. per day of conjugated estrogens in pill form is sufficient. Other estrogens listed in Table 1 are also available by pill.

For vaginal atrophy, direct application of hormone cream to the skin of the vagina solves the problem with the smallest circulating (in the blood stream) quantity of hormone. In fact, vaginally administered estrogen creams relieve symptoms of atrophic vaginitis and hot flashes at all doses tested.[26] The test doses include the newly refined lower dose suggestions via vaginal cream (1.25 mg. of Premarin or .2 mg. of Estrace). Sublingual tablets also work effectively at low doses (.5 mg. every other day).

And estrogen creams also reverse atrophic (deteriorating) urogenital changes.[4]

Premarin is the hormone cream that published studies have most thoroughly evaluated since this brand is the most widely sold hormone therapy in the United States. Other brands that contain the same ingredients should prove to be interchangeable, however. The dose of 1.25 mg. in cream form seems to be fully effective. Lower doses may be safer and can be achieved by using the cream on alternate nights or a fraction of an applicator quantity each night. Estrace, in vaginal cream or sublingual tablet, has also been well studied and shown to be effective. But just about every hormone regimen tested has been shown to be effective in relieving menopausal distress provided the dose is correct. The decision that you and your physician reach, should you opt for hormones, requires a careful consideration of which route (the pill, the tablet, the cream) to select.

Pills, creams, or tablets: which is best for you?

Although adverse side effects of hormone replacement therapy are rare, each should be understood by anyone considering hormones: (1) overstimulation of the liver; (2) increases in blood pressure; and (3) overstimulation of the endometrium, which can (under some but usually not other conditions) induce endometrial hyperplasia.

If you take estrogens by mouth, your liver will receive a higher dose of hormone than if you take HRT by one of the other routes. Why? Consider the route that oral hormones travel: through the mouth, digestive tract (stomach and intestines) and their absorption across the walls of the intestine into the blood stream heading directly for the liver. It is easy to see that the liver is receiving a highly concentrated dose of hormone in comparison with what it would have received if the hormones had been secreted by the ovary. In the natural condition of hormone secretion during the cycling years, estrogen is produced in the ovary and then enters the ovarian vein, travels through the venous return to the heart, enters the lung region, returns to the heart, enters the general arterial circulation, and finally arrives at the liver much watered down. However, when you take estrogens orally, your liver receives a highly concentrated dose of estrogen. You might think of it in the following way. Pour five one-quart bottles of club soda into a tub, add 1.25 mg. of estrogen, and stir. That is approximately how concentrated the estrogen would be in your blood by the time it reached the liver if your ovaries had secreted the estrogen or if your vaginal walls absorbed a dose of estrogen cream. In contrast, dump the 1.25 mg. of estrogen directly into your liver. When you take estrogen by pill, the liver seems to get it fully concentrated before it has had a chance to be diluted. Hence the danger from oral estrogens is that the liver receives a heavier concentration of the hormones than when the ovary is producing them. The studies describing liver overstimulation when hormones are taken by mouth suggest that it is best to avoid taking hormones in pill form unless doses are very low (for oral conjugated estrogens, .6 mg. or less). Although it very rarely occurs, the liver can be overtaxed.[16a] Since there are alternatives available in the form of creams and sublingual tablets, these should represent the most conservative choice for the modern hormone therapy candidate.

Your blood pressure may increase, although this is unlikely. Only oral hormone therapy (pills) has caused this problem in the rare cases where it did happen. Here is how. The liver responds quite rapidly to the oral ingestion of hormones. Large increases in certain blood molecules that sometimes increase the risk of hypertension (high blood pressure) are clearly noted.[17] One liver hormone, renin substrate, increases when oral estrogens are ingested.[28] Renin substrate does not increase in women who take their estrogen by means of vaginal cream, and this is one reason why the cream is a safer route of hormone administration. In young women who take oral contraceptives these renin-substrate increases have been associated with hypertension. In menopausal women the increases in renin substrate have not caused hypertension. Nonetheless, the very rapid response to oral hormones by the liver is cause for caution.

In addition to the liver effects, one can also overstimulate the endometrium of the uterus, a condition that on rare occasions predisposes the uterus to cancer. The resulting hyperplasia is a condition in which the endometrium is stimulated to build up a thick layer of tissue, much like that which a cycling woman produces each month before menstruation takes it away. Although the cancer issue is dealt with in the next chapter, it's appropriate to suggest now the best hormone therapy plan to avoid this risk: you can (1) apply estradiol cream vaginally, because lower doses are effective when taken vaginally; (2) apply estriol cream vaginally; (3) take sublingual wafers whose estradiol gets converted to estrone (E1) once it reaches the blood stream; or (4) take oral estrogen with at least ten days of progesterone opposition for each cycle. The term "progesterone opposition" refers to the mimicking by HRT of a cycling woman's pattern of estrogen plus progesterone. Estrogen naturally stimulates the growth of many tissues; progesterone opposes this stimulation, thereby balancing the estrogen and preventing it from overstimulating tissue development. More on the subject of progesterone will be found in the next chapter.

The two nonoral pill routes of estrogen administration appear equally safe for endometrial (the cancer-prone) tissue, provided the doses you use are not excessively high.

If you take hormones in cream form to reverse vaginal atrophy, you can use less hormone to get the same relief because the sensitive tissues are getting the needed dose before dilution. For those women who are annoyed with the vaginal messiness of a hormone cream preparation, a third method of taking hormones is available. You can place a wafer under your tongue every other day. The wafer will dissolve and be absorbed into your blood stream in less than two minutes. Very low doses (.5 mg. per day) are able to eliminate or severly reduce the hot flashes and vaginal distress characteristic of estrogen deficiencies.[5]

The sublingual wafer is better than oral (pill) estrogen because it does not lead to heavy saturation of estrogen in the liver. By being absorbed into the blood stream first, as in vaginal administration, the liver receives only a diluted dose of estrogen as the blood perfuses that organ. The sublingual wafer is less preferable to the vaginal cream because (1) some of the wafer probably gets swallowed and passes into the digestive track en route to the liver, and (2) it delivers a lower dose to the vaginal tissues than direct administration at the vagina would provide. In order to effectively relieve the vaginal symptoms of menopausal distress, the vaginal application of hormone requires the least powerful dose (.2 mg. every day or every other day), the sublingual wafer the next lowest dose (.5 mg. every other day),[5] and the pill the most powerful dose (1.25 or .625 mg. per day). Lower doses are preferable because the endometrium is less likely to be overstimulated.

What about progesterone?

While estrogen appears to produce a variety of feminizing effects, from breast development to skin suppleness, progesterone functions differently. Progesterone is an important part of a safe hormone-replacement-therapy regimen. The hormone does not appear to play a role in the development of menopausal symptoms the way that estrogen declines have been shown to do. Progesterone does play a role in limiting the tendency of estrogen to produce excess tissue stimulation. Chapter 6 details this role.

Summary

Estrogen relieves the symptoms of menopausal distress, promotes well-being, may facilitate cardiovascular health, prevents or halts bone degeneration, and may even positively affect one's natural immune responses. How often you take the hormone depends on the route of administration, the strength of the dosage, the symptom relief, the presence or absence of progestin in your plan, and other factors. There are many different regimens that are being used successfully. An individual plan can best be worked out by means of cooperation between yourself and your health-care professional.

Endometrial cancer remains the key reservation to the use of HRT at the menopause. Before one begins a hormone replacement regimen, a consideration of the value of progesterone in that therapeutic plan is essential. Progesterone, in addition to the estrogen, is so important in preventing and combatting the risk of endometrial cancer that it must, sensibly, be dealt with in a chapter of its own—the next chapter.

In 1983 the *Journal of the American Medical Association* published a study of estrogen use and all-cause mortality. Two thousand two hundred sixty-nine white women had been followed for six years. The results were that estrogen users had a lower incidence of any kind of death than nonusers. Oophorectomized women who took hormones had only 12 percent the incidence of death than oophorectomized women who took no hormones; hysterectomized women who took hormones had only 34 percent the incidence of death as hysterectomized women who took no hormones; and intact women who took hormones had half the risk of intact women who took no hormones.[6a]

6 / Hormone Replacement Therapy II

THE CANCER RISK

Cancer is scary. If it is unchecked, it can kill you. So can walking across the street. We don't stay inside in order to avoid being killed by a passing car, but we do not take walks along the freeway either. We ought not to avoid hormones before evaluating how low the risks are when proper hormone doses are taken. And make no mistake about it. With new regimens whose doses are lower than regimens that were common ten years ago, the risks, too, are low and must be balanced against the benefits to bone and cardiovascular health which hormones provide. When the first reports came out in 1975 showing an association between cancer of the endometrium and estrogen replacement therapy, the signs were ominous. But the publicity tended to obscure the facts, and in certain crucial ways the general public was misled and left uninformed. More recent studies have shown that while high doses of estrogen do, over time, tend to affect endometrial health adversely, there are alternative courses of treatment available which include (1) lower doses of estrogen and (2) adding progesterone supplements to counterbalance the negative effects that too much estrogen sometimes causes. Both of these approaches radically alter the risks of developing endometrial cancer.

Endometrial cancer

At a simple level, cancer can be understood as an aberrant cellular growth reproducing itself in your body, eating up and replacing healthy cells with malignant ones and destroying tissues as it voraciously spreads and forms tumors. Surgery can often remove tumors. The greater danger lies in their tendency to spread. Little pieces of the tumor break off and spread much like the seeds of a dandelion are dispersed across a great field thanks to the help of a gust of wind. In the case of the tumor, the blood stream serves as the wind, spreading the pieces to other parts of the body.

Your endometrium is a gland lining the central cavity of the uterus. It is pictured on page 78. The endometrium grows and thickens with each menstrual cycle, finally sloughing off during the menstrual flow. This tissue sometimes develops an overgrowth (hyperplasia) or, rarely, the more diseased state—the cancer.

How common and serious is it?

On average, one woman in one thousand per year is diagnosed as having endometrial cancer.[48] Other diseases hit menopausal women more frequently: fourteen per thousand die each year of cardiovascular attacks;[47] more also die each year after hip fracture induced by osteoporosis. The average age of detection for endometrial cancer is about sixty. Seventy percent of the cases occur between fifty and seventy years of age,[34] although en-

dometrial cancer does strike women from twenty-one and older.
It appears to be a slow-growing cancer. The earlier it is detected, the better the cure rate; and close to 90 percent of the
earliest cases are cured. In contrast, the more developed cases
have a poor prognosis. Only 32 percent of these cancer patients
survive the next five years. While advanced stages of endometrial
cancer are very bad, early stages are much less life-threatening.
Moreover, it is reasonable to assume from our current knowledge
of reproductive physiology that before such an early-stage cancer
occurs, there is a long—more than a twelve-month—progression
of hyperplasias. Furthermore, these hyperplasias appear in response to high doses of unopposed estrogen (that is, estrogen
taken without progesterone). You can take progesterone (which
opposes the estrogen influence on endometrial tissue) to avoid
being in such an at-risk category.

How does it develop?

Before the cells reach a state that can be called cancerous, they
appear to pass through several abnormal but noncancerous stages.

There are three stages of increasingly more severe abnormality
of endometrial hyperplasia.[3, 8, 10] The conditions appear to be
progressive in that the earlier stages always precede the development of the later ones.

The first stage is called *cystic hyperplasia,* the second is called
adenomatous hyperplasia, and the third is called *atypical hyperplasia.* Pathologists can, with a microscope, look at slides on
which smears of endometrial tissue have been placed to distinguish one stage of hyperplasia from the next. They employ seven
criteria:

1. the appearance of the glands. The glands become progressively more swollen and enlarged and begin to show overcrowd-
ing.

2. the number of cells per slide. Cystic hyperplasia shows counts of about 100 cells per slide while the more severe, atypical hyperplasia shows about double this number.

3. the number of clumps of cells per slide. Milder conditions show, on average, fewer cell groups, per slide.

4. the average cell size. This gets larger with increasing hyperplastic severity.

5. the average size of the cell nuclei. With increasing severity the area gets larger.[37]

6. increased number of mitotic figures, indicative of increased cell multiplication.

7. variations in the size and the staining properties of the cell nuclei. They may look darker (or lighter) than usual under the microscope.

If the hyperplasia increases in severity, it may develop into endometrial cancer.[14, 37] From a superficial cancer, it can spread into the uterus or into another part of the body by means of the circulatory or lymphatic system. Once in another part of the body, a lump or discrete tumor can form.

How likely is it that cystic glandular hyperplasia will develop into endometrial cancer? It appears to be very unlikely. In one study of 544 premenopausal women with cystic glandular hyperplasia (which were traced and followed for up to twenty-four years), less than 1 percent of the women ever developed endometrial cancer.[29] Figures of this kind are unavailable for hyperplasia at menopause, but the available percentages suggest that cancer rarely develops even in a woman whose endometrium becomes cystic. Adenomatous hyperplasia is much more dangerous.[14]

When endometrial cancer does develop, it is diagnosed according to grade and to stage—from the lowest of I to the highest of

IV. The more clearly defined the tumor(s) is (are), the lower the grade that is assigned. Staging of the tumor from a low of I to a high of IV is also assigned. The higher number denotes a greater size and degree of involvement that the body is experiencing with respect to the malignancies. Cancer cells, unlike benign tumor cells, invade your own tissue and metastasize (spread, like the seeds of a dandelion). The dangerous higher grading (grade IV) denotes that the cancer is no longer neatly isolated in clumps but rather has changed into an undifferentiated state much like pepper sprinkled on eggs. A low-grade cancerous tumor can be identified and removed—usually without further trouble. A higher-grade, less differentiated tumor apparently spreads easier, metastasizing to other parts of the body, where new tumors can form. This is where the greatest danger lies—when a cancer spreads by blood or lymph circulation.

Once a diagnosis of cancer of the uterus has been made, the stage and grade it is assigned helps predict how curable it is. Low-grade and early-stage cancers are almost always curable.[32, 33, 34]

What are the symptoms?

The most common symptom that brings women with endometrial cancer to medical attention is abnormal (that is, unexpected) vaginal bleeding.[32] Not all abnormal bleeding indicates a cancerous condition. But if you are bleeding abnormally, it is important for you to see your physician.[9, 42] Both endometrial hyperplasia and endometrial cancer can exist without any telltale bleeding to signal their presence.[1, 3] However, this is rare.[1, 42] You may have apparent symptoms and most likely not have a disease, or (much less often) you may even have a disease but not have symptoms. Speedy diagnosis and treatment can save life and health.

How is your endometrium examined?

In order to define the state of the endometrium, one must remove cells from it. One cannot use vaginal cells as a way of estimating the state of the endometrial cells.[2, 26, 27] One must examine the endometrial cells which line the uterus. Once the cells are retrieved, they are smeared onto glass slides and studied under a microscope by pathologists.

Several methods are available for retrieving endometrial cells. The older, conventional method was a D & C—dilatation (expanding the opening of the cervix) and curettage (using a spoon-like instrument to scrape a bit of tissue from the lining of the uterus). "Cell samplers," an alternative method to D & C for obtaining endometrial cells, are simpler, faster, and avoid anesthesia. One of several cell samplers currently available is used: the Garcia Endometrial Curette (developed by Celso-Ramón García),[37] the Isaacs Endometrial Cell Sampler,[21] or the Endopap. Each is pictured in Figures 14, 15, and 16.

The cell sampler is introduced into the vagina, and the narrower end passes through the opening of the cervix to reach the walls of the endometrium. The cervical stop prevents any other part of the instrument from gaining entry into the uterus. If you have a narrow cervix, the Isaacs Cell Sampler will stretch it as it penetrates through the narrow opening (os) to the womb. This stretching open of the narrow cervical canal can be uncomfortable. The Endopap, because it is thinner, does not cause this discomfort. Likewise, the Garcia Curette is gentler. Once the cell sampler has gained entry into the uterus, some of the endometrial cells are removed, either by a gentle scraping (the Endopap or the Garcia Curette) or by using a syringe attached to hollow end of the shield (Isaacs Cell Sampler or Garcia Curette). The syringe is illustrated on the Isaacs Cell Sampler and would be attached, in the same way, to the Garcia Curette. The head of the syringe

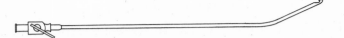

Figure 14 The Garcia Endometrial Curette

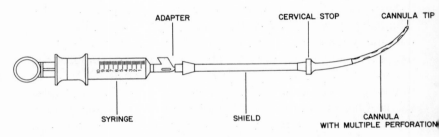

Figure 15 The Isaacs Endometrial Cell Sampler

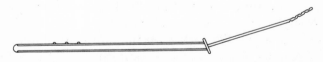

Figure 16 The Endopap

is manipulated to create a vacuum. This vacuum causes some of the cells from the endometrium to be sucked back into the sampler. Very few women find this alternative to D & C more than "slightly uncomfortable."[21] The Endopap does not provide as much tissue and therefore is more limited to screening (rather than diagnostic) techniques. Studies comparing the accuracy of diagnosis between conventional D & C and the diagnostic endometrial suction curettage support that both produce adequate tissue for accurate diagnoses.[4] More recent studies suggest that vacuum curettage has increased the accuracy of diagnosis over the D & C.[44] The suction curettage (either Isaac or Garcia form) has the advantage of avoiding the necessity for dilating the cervix (as in a D & C). It is faster—it takes less than three minutes. This way, any hyperplasias (should they be present) can be detected at the most curable stage. The suction curettage requires no anesthetics, thereby avoiding those risks.

Who is at risk for endometrial cancer?

Endometrial cancer patients are more likely to be obese, nulliparous (never have had a baby), hypertensive (have high blood pressure), and to have taken high doses of unopposed estrogen treatment for a long duration.[9] The least critical factor turns out to be the estrogen, although it gets the most publicity.

The greatest risk for endometrial cancer appears to be obesity. Usually this is defined as being more than 30 percent overweight.[15] One research group compared patients with endometrial cancer to aged-matched healthy women for a thirty-year period. Obesity turned out to be the best predictor of endometrial cancer. Obesity accounted for much more cancer than did nulliparity (never having given birth), and nulliparity accounted for much more cancer than did estrogen use. Another thirty-year study of 1,590 cases of uterine cancer found that a startling 51 percent of the cancer victims were obese.[35] If you are very overweight, you would be wise to monitor your endometrial health

carefully. Have either regular (annual) endometrial checkups—
(endometrial biopsy) or take the Progestin Challenge Test, described later in this chapter.

If you are short (5 feet 1 inch or less) and obese, the risks have
been shown to be less since these risks apply predominantly to
taller women. The tallest women, those over 5 feet 6 inches, are
taking the biggest cancer risk if they become obese.[31, 54] We do
not know why. With regard to your weight, one other point is
worth noting. Slender women who take estrogen may be at a
higher risk than other women who take estrogen for a different
reason. As described earlier, your fat cells actively convert androstenedione (an abundant menopausal hormone secreted by the
adrenals and the aging ovaries) into estrone. The more fat you
have, the higher your estrone level is likely to be. Thin women
have, on average, lower levels of estrogen and, consequently, may
suffer greater menopausal distress than heavier women. They may
overcompensate with a dose of estrogen treatment that is dispro-
portionately high for their small body size. Currently, hormone
dosages are not prescribed with considerations of a woman's size
—but they probably should be.

Being nulliparous also places women in the higher-risk category
for endometrial cancer.[31, 35] It was shown that having had even
one child sharply reduces the risk for endometrial cancer.[31] Apparently, the endometrium changes in some unknown way after
it has supported a growing fetus and placenta to make the development of a uterine cancer less likely.

Hypertension is the third most critical risk factor.[35] Almost
half of the endometrial cancer patients have diastolic blood pressures of more than 100 mm. Hg. Normal values should be around
60 to 80. But it is not clear which comes first—high blood pressure or endometrial cancer.

Do hormones cause cancer?

Estrogen is one critical hormone controlling the growth of the endometrium during each cycle. Estrogen therapy at menopause likewise influences the growth of the lining. Too much estrogen can lead to overgrowth. High doses of estrogen have, not surprisingly, been shown to be associated with endometrial overgrowth (hyperplasia).[3, 5, 12, 20, 23, 24, 40, 55] This overgrowth looks like the beginning growth of cancer. The biomedical research community is not agreed on whether hyperplasia and cancer are directly connected or separate entities. In any case, there is evidence that high doses of unopposed estrogen predispose some women to endometrial cancer. Unfortunately, when the first reports appeared and caused such a scare, they failed to point out that it was high, not low, doses that were largely responsible. High doses of unopposed estrogen produce an unnecessary risk. Even though very few (7 per 1,000) women who take this risk will have a problem, there is no reason for you to gamble, because low doses fully relieve the distressing symptoms of menopause, prevent the devastation of osteoporosis, and do not appear to place you at risk for endometrial cancer.[30] In fact, in one thirty-year study that monitored the women of an entire county in Minnesota, those with endometrial cancer were no more likely to have used low levels of estrogen (less than 1.25 mg. of conjugated oral estrogen) than those without cancer.[30] In that study, just as in the others described, high doses of estrogen *did* increase the risk, as expected. Moreover, by adding progesterone in the proper way you can actively reduce your risk of endometrial cancer to levels below that of women who take no hormones.[11] More about this later.

How much estrogen is too much?

Each drug company packages its estrogen in a series of four to five increasingly more powerful doses. Table 1 on pages 114–115 shows the range of doses for some of the more common kinds of estrogen currently being sold. Your doctor can show you the guidebook he or she uses and go over with you the range of doses of the particular brand he or she selects for you. The *Physicians' Desk Reference*, published yearly, is one such text. You might even find it in your local library or at the book store. While it is not a complete compendium of drugs, it does reflect the information that is found in drug package inserts. These are required by the Food and Drug Administration. For example, as of 1982 for Premarin (a current best seller) the pill form comes in doses as low as .3 mg. per day of estrogen and ranges upward to .625 mg., 1.25 mg., and 2.5 mg. For vaginal cream, the low dose begins with .3 mg. per day when one-eighth of the applicator capacity is used. The total cream applied each day to yield this low dose of estrogen is one-half a gram's worth. Clearly, the lower your dose of estrogen, the better off your endometrium will be. The choice of estrogen dose must reflect a consideration of endometrial safety that is balanced against the benefits that were described in the previous chapter—relief from menopausal symptoms and the improved general health of the skeletal and cardiovascular systems. The more unopposed estrogen you take each day, the greater the risk is that you will overstimulate your endometrium.

What about progesterone?

Progesterone helps prevent or oppose endometrial disease. In fact, the old terminology, ERT, estrogen replacement therapy, began to give way to a newer term, HRT, hormone replacement therapy. This reflected the developing perception that proper replacement therapy included more than just estrogen. Investigators en masse were starting to realize that since the normal cycling woman had a repeating sequence of estrogen plus progesterone, it made sense to mimic this set of ingredients in menopausal replacement programs.

As early as 1974, some investigators were saying that progestogens, in adequate dosages, could reverse hyperplasias that had been induced by estrogen therapies.[41, 51] In 1978 a review of 8,170 women showed that women who took estrogen in combination with progestogens (P) actually had less incidence of endometrial cancer than women who took no hormones. The terms "progestin" and "progestogen" are the names given to any substance with progesterone-like activity. Women who took estrogens (at a time when high doses were common) without progestin had three times the incidence of this cancer than nonhormone users. The actual numbers are as follows:[46]

- In the 2,088 estrogen (E) users, there were 8 cancers—3.8 per 1,000.

- In 1,515 untreated women, there were 13 cancers—1.6 per 1,000.

- In 775 users of other hormones, there was 1 cancer—1.3 per 1,000.

- In the 3,792 E + P users, there was 1 cancer—.3 per 1,000.

In another study, long-term E users (five or more years) were compared with nonusers to show that while estrogen alone did increase the risk of endometrial cancer, progesterone protected against this cancer. No cancer appeared in any of the patients treated with progestogen supplements.[17] Other studies showed the same thing.[3, 9, 11]

The influence of progesterone on endometrial tissue has been studied by molecular biologists. They have shown that progesterone acts on endometrial tissue in such way that the endometrium ceases its usual ability to grow in response to estrogen.[6, 13, 25, 43] The literature on this issue is consistent. Unopposed high doses of estrogens may be dangerous; low doses of estrogens (e.g., .625 mg. per day of Premarin) are usually not harmful; and the influence of progesterone on endometrial health is good—even reverting hyperplastic tissue back to normal.[8]

How should progesterone be taken?

Once it was appreciated that progesterone is an important part of a conservative hormone replacement program, doctors asked: How much progesterone should be taken and for how many days each month? The earliest report, in 1966, was by Dr. Georgeanna Seegar Jones, a pioneer in female endocrinology. She went on record saying: "The most effective hormonal support can be given by the administration of a progestogen in combination with estrogen for 20 days each month. If hysterectomy has been carried out, continuous estrogen therapy is quite satisfactory."[22] Dr. Robert Greenblatt of the Medical College of Georgia was another early pioneer in progestin therapy.

The studies that compared the reduction in risk of cancer as a function of progesterone use did not have available to them women taking progesterone for as many days as Dr. Jones had recommended. Those few physicians who were prescribing progesterone tended to limit its use to five or six days out of each month. Even when used for five or six days, the beneficial results were unambiguous and startling.[42] More recently, a series of studies make it clear that it is not how much progesterone you take that matters, but how many consecutive days you take it. It's far better to take a little bit each day for ten to thirteen days than to flood your system with a high dose over five to six days.[3, 11, 42, 45]

Although no one has yet rigorously tested Dr. Jones's original suggestion of twenty days of progesterone each month, the direction of the trend suggests that she may be correct. For now, it is recommended that you work out a program with your physician as follows.

If you have an intact uterus and take an estrogen dose over the very minimal level, take a progestogen with this estrogen during the last ten days that you take estrogen each hormone cycle.

Expect to menstruate each month on the days you abstain from the hormones. In effect, you are mimicking nature's hormonal cycle, and a menstrual-like flow often occurs when hormones (estrogen and progesterone) are temporarily stopped for the last week of each month. If three months on this routine pass and no menstrual-like flow ensues, you can eliminate the progestogen from your program.[9, 11] In medical language, your endometrium was "challenged" with progestin and did not respond (with a menstrual flow). If no menstrual period follows on the hormone-free days, you can assume that your endometrium is okay—that is, it was not in a state of overstimulation due to the unopposed estrogen you had been taking[11]—and, therefore, you can avoid the progesterone for another six months. You should then reintroduce progesterone and repeat the challenge test. If the challenge is met with a menstrual-like bleeding, continue the progestogen until three cycles pass without bleeding. The bleeding after the challenge is good for you. It represents a sloughing off of the endometrial tissue that had been building up in response to the estrogen therapy. This "Progestin Challenge Test" is a useful way of monitoring your endometrium without endometrial examination and has been shown to be remarkably effective at preventing endometrial cancers.[11] For women who are obese and not taking hormones, this Progestin Challenge Test provides a useful way of reducing the risk of undetected cancer. If you are heavy, you also would be wise to discuss this precaution with your physician even if you are not taking HRT.

Several forms of progestins are available in pill form, with variations in the package doses occurring from one country to the next. Appropriately taken, each seems to prevent the development of a hyperplastic endometrium. The recommended procedure is to take progestin for at least ten days during each cycle.[18] Four different chemical forms of progestin are commonly in use today: norethindrone, norethindrone acetate, medroxyprogesterone acetate, and norgestrel. The recommended dosage has been set at 5 mg. of norethindrone acetate or 10 mg. of medroxyprogesterone acetate, but the receptor studies just coming out suggest that lower doses may provide equal protection. In all probability, the effective doses will soon be shown to be 1 mg. of norethindrone acetate, 2 mg. of medroxyprogesterone acetate, or 150 micrograms of D/L norgestrel per day during each of the last ten to thirteen days that you take the estrogens.[50, 51, 52] These dosages are about one-fifth the dosages first tried, and the newest studies suggest that these low doses protect the endometrium fully. Women taking higher doses of progestin sometimes report some initial discomfort the first few months—premenstrual tension, a bloated feeling, or some menstrual cramping. These symptoms usually vanish by the fourth month. The lower doses may turn out to have no side effects at all, but the question is still being studied.

The doses mentioned above are from studies in Great Britain, where the progestins are packaged a little differently than in the United States. In the United States norethindrone acetate is supplied as a 5 mg. tablet sold under the brand name of Norlutate. Norethindrone, which according to its manufacturer is about half as potent a progestin as norethindrone acetate, is sold as a 5 mg. tablet marketed as Norlutin and is also available as a .35 mg. tablet sold as Micronor. The 5 mg. tablets are scored so that they can be broken into two doses of 2.5 mg. each. Medroxyprogesterone acetate is packaged under the name of Provera by one company (but is also manufactured under the names Curetab and Amen by two others),[7] and is supplied as a 2.5 mg. tablet and as a 10 mg. tablet. Norgestrel is marketed under the name Ovrette and is available in .075 mg. tablets. With the help of your doctor you can decide what kind of progestin and how much of it is right for you. The research clearly shows that ten to thirteen days per month is the most appropriate length of time to take the progestin.[28, 36]

If hormones are so great, why aren't all doctors prescribing them?

Hormone replacement therapy is riddled with controversy, and the medical textbooks which guide physicians and medical students are sometimes not current about menopause research. For example, one widely used medical physiology textbook in its 1981 version[16] had this hopelessly outdated "factual information" to offer about menopausal symptoms and treatments:

These symptoms are of sufficient magnitude in approximately 15% of women to warrant treatment. If psychotherapy fails, daily administration of an estrogen in small quantities will reverse the symptoms, and, by gradually decreasing the dose the postmenopausal woman is likely to avoid severe symptoms; unfortunately such treatment prolongs the symptoms. (p. 1016)

The clear implication is that psychotherapy should be the first treatment of choice for a woman's menopausal symptoms. This guidance flies in the face of our current knowledge of the relationship between changing hormone levels and the appearance of menopausal symptoms. Moreover, the recommendation that women taking hormones should be gradually weaned from them does not take into account the fact that when this is done a woman may risk the development of osteoporosis.

Conclusion

Ultimately, it is you who reaps the benefits that hormone therapy provides. It is you, not your doctor, who must make an "informed" choice about what benefits and risks you will accept. Specific conditions that can allow for hormones but that require a careful consideration and more frequent checkups include a past history of any hormone-dependent cancer or pelvic disease (like fibroids or endometriosis). Gall-bladder disease also requires a careful medical monitoring. If you decide to take hormones with such a history, then any symptoms of pain or uncontrolled bleeding will probably cause your physician to take you off hormone therapy. Likewise, if you have high blood pressure, diabetes, varicose veins, smoke heavily, or are more than 30 percent over your proper weight, you may decide it is best to forgo hormone therapy, although many women who have these conditions can safely enjoy hormone therapy with careful medical care.

There has been considerable question about cystic breasts and hormone use. Several studies have explored relationships with respect to cystic breasts, HRT, and breast cancer. Some information is available. Women whose breasts become cystic while taking HRT may be at a slightly increased risk of developing breast cancer: but according to several studies, this risk is only found in the users of *higher* doses of *unopposed* estrogen (more than .625 mg. of conjugated estrogen).[19, 39] Moreover, some investigators have concluded, after studying several thousand menopausal women, that postmenopausal estrogen use can neither be indicted as causing nor considered to prevent breast cancer.[39] However, in a 1982 report of a large sample of menopausal women, when breast cancer did develop, HRT users fared better. In this study, women who were taking hormones had half the risk of death as women who were not taking hormones.[7, 8] In a similar fashion to the discoveries of the protective effect of progestins on endometrial cancer, recent information (studies completed but not yet published) supports that breast tissue is also protected by progestins. More information will undoubtably be obtained in the next five years. For now, if you are at risk for cystic breasts, progestin opposition should probably be included into a low-dose estrogen regimen, should you opt for HRT. You should not take hormones if you have any of the following diseases: undiagnosed vaginal bleeding, acute vascular thrombosis (sudden onset blockage of blood vessels), neuro-ophthalmologic vascular disease (diseases of the blood vessels in the visual system), breast cancer, or high blood pressure that resulted from hormone replacement therapy.

In any case, you should know that there is a risk whenever you take a medication. No one knows for sure what the effects will be for a specific person. You must weight the risks (low though they be) against the benefits (which are many and significant) and choose the alternative best suited to you. Every experience in life carries with it some risk. Walking across a busy street, exerting oneself in a strenuous game of tennis, driving or riding in a car, and so forth carry risks of death from internal or external accident. From the abundance of rigorously designed studies, the increased risks of properly dosed hormones appear to be lower than any of the ones just listed, provided that you are not in the "should not take hormones" category. And for those of you in the "careful consideration" category, you must carefully weigh the risk against the benefit.

With the clear understanding of the benefits of a low-dose estrogen or a moderate-dose estrogen program with progesterone added to it, you have the knowledge to make an intelligent choice. Although the medical community has accepted the responsibility for health care of society, the individuals have the final responsibility for their own health care. To do this effectively requires motivation, the willingness to take responsibility for themselves, and knowledge. You must initiate and maintain that motivation to establish your best possible health. This does not mean that you do not need the help that your physician can provide. Rather, you can use the information in this book to help you work *with* a health care professional in order to maximize your own proper care.

Summary

Taking too much estrogen can lead to overgrowth of the endometrium and may increase the risk of developing endometrial cancer. But, according to the best studies available, relatively low doses of estrogen relieve menopausal symptoms and prevent the development of osteoporosis without causing a woman to risk endometrial cancer. Moreover, taking progestogen in combination with estrogen—in effect mimicking the body's natural hormone cycle—appears to reduce the risk of getting endometrial cancer when compared with taking no hormones at all. In any decision about taking ovarian hormones, endometrial safety should be a major consideration. Your doctor can help you decide what kind of a program is right for you. Although there are women who, for a variety of reasons, should not take hormones, if you are like most menopausal women, you can have the benefits of hormone replacement therapy without compromising endometrial safety.

7/ Sexuality in the Menopausal Years

I personally have had a satisfying relationship with my husband. He is very much in love with me and requires a lot of sexual attention. Almost every other night. I think, because of all this affection, I am a very contented female. His appetite hasn't changed at all, but he has become more tolerant of my disinterest many nights. I enjoy sex, find it more of an effort to reach orgasm, but can if I put my mind to it. I don't crave it. I have many activities and work every day, and constant worries about my 2 grown daughters (one who has been very ill) that drain my efforts to concentrate more on bedtime romance. . . . I am 51.

I obtain less satisfaction from sex and find myself making more excuses as to not have sex. I am 51 years old.

The complexity of human sexuality and the diversity of human sexual experience is clearly evident in the comments of different menopausal women.

If you have the good fortune to have a partner you value, sex can be one of the most pleasurable experiences that life has to offer. There is comfort to be had in being held and caressed. Erotic pleasure takes many forms unique to each individual. At every age it can be wonderful. But our society tends to be youth-oriented, and it is easy to get the idea that sex is only for the young. Then, too, many people equate sex with reproduction and believe that the end of a woman's reproductive years brings a decline of sexual desire and pleasure. While these notions are by no means universally true, it is natural enough for you to wonder about your own sexuality during menopause. Is there a difference in sexual appetite? How does the change of life affect your capacity for sexual pleasure?

These are not easy questions to answer because a person's sexual feelings are related to many different things. A sense of health, well-being, and vigor can make you feel sexy. You will probably feel less so if you are flushing, tired, or depressed. What is your attitude toward sex—generally positive or more negative? Have your past sexual experiences been good ones or bad ones? Sexual feelings can be intensified by the presence of an interesting partner and by your partner's interest in you. Each couple forms their own world, and one cannot fully study these deeply personal and private experiences in the same way that one can measure hormones or bone mass. Masters and Johnson, pioneers in the study of the physiology of sexual response, and others since have contributed enormously to our understanding of sexuality. They have shown how the nervous system activates muscular response as well as other physiological changes during sex. But no one has been able to examine adequately the range of individual experience that occurs within the private domain of a man-woman relationship. In physics, the problem is defined by "the Heisenberg Uncertainty Principle." It states, in simplified form, that the tools one must use to measure a dynamic process inevitably disturb and distort the very process one is trying to measure. For this reason investigators are bound to produce "uncertain" results. This chapter reviews the best information that is available on the subjects, but it should be understood that studies of human sexuality have only just begun to explore seriously this most complex area of human experience. And they will, undoubtedly, continue to produce "uncertain" findings.

Changes in frequency

A number of studies have shown that women tend to be less sexually active with the passage of years.[1, 13, 14, 18, 21, 23] The cause may be due to changes in either partner. Consider this comment from a fifty-five-year-old woman:

> *Sex drives and desire for me doesn't change much except that our husbands don't have the same sex drive as before. They perform, but it's not the same—more like a feeling of obligation than an actual drive. It's no wonder so many middle age men leave their wives for younger women—they have to prove to themselves they are still the "macho guy."*

Another fifty-year-old woman simply said:

> *My sex drive has diminished slightly.*

In the Stanford Study 49 percent of the women said that their sexual activity had declined since their menstrual cycles had begun to change; 38 percent reported no change; and 14 percent told of an increase in activity. A variety of reasons were given for the decrease in sex. Some women told of being less interested in sex. Others had found it more difficult to locate a suitable male partner. Some had found new living arrangements that offered them less privacy. Privacy problems tended to diminish the pleasure in sexual encounters and, therefore, to make their occurrence less likely. But some women had found a new love, and these women tended to report an increase in sexual activity—as we would expect. Whatever your particular situation, having knowledge about the physiology of sexual response can help you to understand your own sexuality during the menopause years.

Changes in sexual physiology

In women of reproductive age one of the first signs of sexual arousal is when the walls of the vagina begin to produce droplets of fluid which quickly form a slippery coating throughout the entire vaginal barrel. The same moistening reaction occurs in response to any vaginal irritation, including infection. This response is nature's mechanism for washing out and diluting the contents of the vaginal tract. With the characteristic diminution of estrogen at menopause the vagina is much less moist. In addition, the walls of the vagina become tissue-paper thin and lose some of their ability to lubricate quickly and efficiently in response to sexual arousal. So even if you feel yourself becoming aroused, it may take several minutes before your vagina catches up and begins to lubricate. The hormone declines of menopause also cause the vagina to become smaller (shorter and narrower) and lose some of its elasticity. Vaginal dryness and a decrease in elasticity can make intercourse painful—a condition known as *dyspareunia*.

Thick vaginal walls serve as kind of a cushion during intercourse, protecting the bladder and the urethra from the pressure that is produced by the thrusting of an erect penis. With the loss of this cushion, it is fairly common for intercourse to be followed by a strong urge to urinate. Some menopausal women also complain of a burning sensation during urination that persists for several days after a long session of intercourse.[19, 20]

In women of all ages the experience of orgasm is accompanied by strong contractions of the uterus. Lacking sufficient estrogen, the uterus of a menopausal woman shrinks, and for some the uterine contractions during orgasm can be painful. One woman over sixty described the contractions as being "almost like labor pains except that they occur more rapidly."[20] We do not know the reason for this pain but suspect that it is related to hormone deficiencies because of the timing of its appearance.

Even women who have never had any discomfort during sexual activity before menopause may begin to experience some degree of distress as the hormone diminution of the change of life progresses. Not surprisingly, estrogen therapy improves vaginal lubrication in menopausal women.[5, 22] Some menopausal women taking estrogen also report a significant improvement in sexual interest, activity, satisfaction, experience of pleasure, sexual fantasy, and capacity for orgasm.[8, 11] But other studies do not find this to be true.[25] According to Masters and Johnson, HRT with both estrogen and progesterone is necessary in order to eliminate the discomfort that some women experience from orgasmic uterine contractions. Neither hormone used by itself will relieve complaints of this kind.[19, 20] Perhaps this therapy may be of some help; and if you are having this problem, you may want to discuss this with your doctor. But he or she may not have a ready answer for you because the issue has not yet been rigorously researched.

Not every woman is affected in the same way by the change of life; not every woman needs HRT. In some menopausal women the ovaries and/or adrenal glands continue to produce sufficient estrogen so that there are few, if any, menopausal symptoms. In such women, the vagina retains much of its tone and natural appearance and continues to lubricate during sexual arousal in a pattern characteristic of a younger woman.[19]

Although vaginal dryness is a frequent complaint of menopausal women, Masters and Johnson[19, 20] note an interesting exception. They found that three women in their study—each one over sixty years old—lubricated rapidly when aroused. These women had continued to have sex on a regular basis (once to twice per week) all through their adult lives. The facility with which these women lubricated is particularly remarkable because, in each case, their vaginal skin had atrophied to the tissue-paper thinness characteristic of other menopausal women. Why were they exceptions? Note what one fifty-year-old woman in Philadelphia had to say:

My friends complain about how dry they have become and resort to lubricants. I never had any such problem. I attribute it to the fact that through my husband's efforts and insistence, I am still sexually active.

Regular sexual activity may promote the capacity for rapid vaginal lubrication and in this respect counteract at least one of the effects of a paucity of estrogen. Regular sexual activity may have other beneficial effects. Data from the Stanford study show that women approaching menopause who have regular weekly sexual intercourse tend to be either entirely free of hot flashes or experience milder ones than women who either abstain from sexual activity or have more sporadic sexual activity.[6] They also show higher levels of estrogen and a tendency to maintain this level as the months pass. In contrast, the sporadic and celibate women had lower levels of estrogen and, three months later, had lost an additional 10 percent in their estrogen concentration.

Hormones and sexual desire

If the walls of your vagina have thinned and you have trouble lubricating, intercourse can be uncomfortable and even painful. Are you flashing, itching, and depressed? All of these common symptoms of menopause may lessen your interest in sex. These symptoms are relieved by estrogen, and this may be one reason why some menopausal women report an improvement in sexual desire after starting HRT.[8] The capacity for reaching a comfortable orgasm and for achieving a feeling of sexual satisfaction are also improved among menopausal women taking hormones.[8, 11]

Hormones may even have a direct effect on sexual interest. Many women experience a loss of sexual desire around the time of menopause.[9] Some, wanting to avoid hormone therapy but hoping to increase their libido, try vitamin E. But according to well-designed research investigations,[12] vitamin E does not affect libido. In the Stanford Menopause Study a third of the women, all of whom were well into their menopausal transition, reported a recent definite decline in sexual desire. Scientists do not know the precise relationship between hormones and sexual desire in women because the necessary research studies have not yet been done. Desire is clearly related to factors other than one's underlying level of sexual interest. The availability of an interesting and interested sexual partner is obviously relevant, and the influence of hormones on desire may be relatively modest in comparison with these and other social influences. As one forty-seven-year-old sexually interested woman from California put it when describing her recent sexual history:

One romance 2 years ago—but there are no men available! Sad—sad!

Two recent studies did show that hormones and sexual interest are linked in some women.[2, 10] Women (twenty-one to thirty-seven years) with regular menstrual cycles showed the highest incidence of "autosexual" activities during the middle of their cycles. The autosexual activities included masturbation, sexually arousing fantasies, dreams, and so on. These women were also more likely to initiate love-making with their partner during the middle of their cycles. It seems, therefore, that sexual desire was peaking during the middle of the menstrual cycle. This is the time of the month when the ovary is secreting high levels of estrogen, and for some women testosterone and androstenedione levels are maximal then also. In some way that we do not yet fully understand, these hormones may increase sexual desire. Since the middle of the cycle, around the time of ovulation, is the time when intercourse is most likely to result in pregnancy, a pattern of this kind is sensible from a survival perspective. Organisms that are motivated to have sex when they are fertile will be the ones that have offspring; survival of a species requires fertile reproduction. Since ovarian hormones appear to increase sexual desire in at least some women of reproductive age, it is possible (although as yet unconfirmed) that the reverse hormonal condition—the hormone declines of menopause—could lead to the reverse libidinal pattern in some women: a decrease in sexual interest. If you've begun the change of life and notice your interest in sex declining, perhaps this is why.

But not everybody is the same. Some women experience an increase in sexual desire around the time of menopause. A number of reasons can account for the increase. Androgens are still being produced, and there is some evidence that these hormones can stimulate desire.[3, 4, 24] Another factor is cultural change. More and more one hears that we are seeing women in the company of men younger than themselves. Does a younger man stimulate a woman's libido more effectively? It probably depends on the woman as well as the man. Then, too, for many women whose children have grown, there may be more time and energy for sex. The so called "empty-nest syndrome" that sometimes precedes a depression can just as often stimulate a reawakening to new potentials in life. If so, sexual interest can be among these new focus points.

But a word of caution. If you are still having irregular cycles, you are probably still ovulating some of the time and can become pregnant. You should use some form of contraception until you stop menstruating altogether if you want to prevent a pregnancy.

Masturbation

For people of any age, finding a suitable sexual partner isn't easy. If you are alone, you may discover that masturbation is a good way to experience pleasure and discharge sexual tensions. Such activity is common, harmless, and, although no investigator has yet assessed it, may be health-promoting.

A recently published book, *The Hite Report*, devotes thirty-four pages to detailing the different ways women masturbate. Although there has been some controversy about the book, it does contain some valuable information. When women were asked to describe the importance of masturbation in their lives, there was a wide range of answers: it was used as a substitute for successful coitus; it helped prevent one from going "nuts"; it provided health during the times when a partner was not available; it increased one's understanding of one's own body, thereby promoting better sex with another person; it produced a calming effect; and it was an important part of one's own sensuality.[17]

Aging and male sexual physiology

The whole gamut of interpersonal attitudes affect sexual experience. How two people relate to each other is probably much more important than the mechanics of sexual physiology, but it helps to understand the latter. If you have a male partner over fifty, you may well notice that his sexual physiology is changing, too.

For many men, erections occur quickly. For men over fifty it may take longer, and direct stimulation of the penis can become more important. Even with direct stimulation it can take several minutes before an older man's penis becomes really firm. While young men often ejaculate prematurely, older men seldom have this problem. One of the usual things about getting older is that the drive to ejaculate becomes less urgent so that intercourse can last longer. Or the older man may be unable to maintain his erection.

On average as a man gets older, the volume of his ejaculate begins to decrease, and the force with which it is expelled is diminished. After a man ejaculates, his erection softens and there is a waiting period before he will be ready, or even capable, of having another erection of sufficient firmness for intercourse. In a young man this refractory period is usually measured in minutes. For a man over fifty the detumescence can occur much faster, and it may take several hours or more before the capacity for a full erection returns.

Sometimes it happens that a man does not ejaculate in response to sexual intercourse. This does not mean that he cannot continue to ejaculate each time but only that he may come to accept that ejaculation is not nearly as important to his sexual satisfaction as it used to be. Putting it another way, a man in his sixties may continue to have sex eagerly and frequently and to express satisfaction even though he may not ejaculate each time. Every man is different and follows his own time table. Some may be in their forties or fifties when these changes occur. Others may be well into their eighties.

Why do these changes occur? This is a very complex question. They may be the result of a gradually declining level of testosterone or may simply be one of the many consequences of the aging processes or of some other factors that have not yet been quantified. Systematic study of testosterone replacement therapy and sexual functioning in aging males could answer this question, but so far no such studies have been reported. And what's more, testosterone therapy may not be of any value. We do know that, for the vast majority, the decline in testosterone levels parallels the declining frequency of erection.[7] And *very* low levels of androgen have been related to declining sexual function.[4] This is rare. But a decline in a man's level of testosterone with age is not inevitable.[15]

Even in this age of relative sexual enlightenment, it is a popular fallacy that the aging process robs a man of his capacity for sexual pleasure. Few men are immune to fears of losing their sexuality and may view with alarm as a sign of impending sexual failure age-related changes in their sexual activity.[16] Anticipating difficulty at achieving an erection, a man may avoid the expected humiliation of impotence by withdrawing from opportunities for sexual contact. If he has been monogamously attached, he may blame his partner for his difficulty and perhaps seek rejuvenation by having sex with another woman. In the short run, the sexual power of a new relationship may do wonders for his self-esteem and perhaps ease his fears. It could also happen that a man who fears impotence might fail to perform with a new partner, too. In any case, the likelihood is that these changes in a man's sexual capabilities are as natural and as inevitable as the other physical changes of aging. If a man is in good health, however, he could very well retain the capacity for erection and sexual pleasure into his eighties and perhaps beyond.

Age, then, can affect the sexual abilities of your partner. If you view these changes with alarm, it is likely that he will also. As a man ages, the fact that it may take longer to achieve an erection may not mean that he finds you less attractive as a sexual partner. It may only mean that in some instances, in order to get a full erection, it may be necessary for his penis to receive more direct stimulation than when he was younger. Many women feel that they have not satisfied their partner unless intercourse results in his orgasm (ejaculation). You should appreciate that as your partner gets older, he may be adequately satisfied with sex even though he does not have an ejaculation.

Good sex has a lot to do with how well two people communicate. Men and women often find it difficult to talk about what is bothering them, particularly when it comes to issues of physical intimacy. Men in particular, however, sometimes feel that any expression of fear or insecurity on their part will be seen as unmasculine, and they will go to extraordinary lengths to preserve an illusion of confidence and control. The man who acts the most secure may be the one who feels the most insecure. This is unfortunate because talking about one's fears often helps to relieve them. If a relationship is a good one in other respects, sexual problems can probably be resolved; but some effort at communication is required. If communication cannot be achieved without help, counseling is sometimes very effective.

Summary

Menopause need not herald the end of your sexual life. Although some people may, quite happily, choose that route, many others do not. If sex has been important to you as a younger woman, it is likely to continue to be important to you as you approach and pass through your menopause. You will probably notice some changes in your sexual physiology that parallel some of the other changes you are experiencing. This is natural since all of these effects can be traced to the decrease in ovarian hormone output which marks the change of life. Just as HRT alleviates the other symptoms of menopause, the appropriate HRT can prevent (or reverse) the vaginal and uterine atrophy of menopause and help you to continue to have a healthy and satisfying sex life throughout your postmenopausal years. In fact, with the knowledge that comes from experience, your capacity for sensuality can mature as your body does; you may find that the sexual pleasure can easily become better than it ever was before. If you come to experience sex as an expression of love, as a means of building a closeness of relationship, as a means of communicating sharing and caring, as a source of erotic pleasure, as a time for feeling, as a time when problems cease and pleasure is meaningful, as a time of acceptance and being accepted, then aging can be a period of growth. In fact to the mature person, as the body ages, the sexual responses slow and the spirit can grow. Shall you embrace the wisdom of your body? If you slow down and focus on the areas of sexual activity that provide pleasure, full sexual enjoyment can easily become better than it ever was before. After periods of sexual abstinence, you should expect some degree of narrowing and thinning of the vagina as well as a loss of lubrication response. But these problems will disappear if sexual activity is resumed with gentle and limited coital thrusting—and perhaps the use of a lubricant.

8 / Hysterectomy

The removal of a uterus—hysterectomy—requires major surgery. The removal of the ovaries—ovariectomy or oophorectomy
—is commonly performed at the same time. Why? Why are
women in record numbers having these vital organs removed?
Should they? Apparently not always. A physician speaking about
the uterus stated:

> I am unaware of any other important organ that is effec-
> tively removed without first assessing its degree of mal-
> function.[25]

Such highly critical views are being expressed more frequently.
By contrast, fourteen years ago a very different view was expressed
by another gynecologist:

> The uterus has but one function: reproduction. After the
> last planned pregnancy, the uterus becomes a useless,

bleeding, symptom-producing, potentially cancer-bearing organ and therefore should be removed.[67]

Increasing evidence supports the fact that the uterus is anything but useless. Your uterus is a muscular glandular organ, a living, functioning tissue which responds to ovarian hormones. Besides its well-known role in housing a growing fetus, it appears to have other important functions. It responds to certain important hormones. While not life-threatening, hysterectomy may lead to, or even directly produce, certain sexual deficits in some women.[14] If sex is important to you and you are considering having this operation, you will need to also consider the possible effects of the operation on your sex life.[14, 43]

Your ovaries also serve very vital functions throughout your life. Remember that in a modified way your ovaries continue to secrete important hormones even though you might have passed your reproductive years. Even when you must lose your uterus, your ovaries can continue to serve you well.

How many women are having hysterectomies?

Since 1962, the incidence of hysterectomy has been rising in the United States. In 1962 about 31 percent of the menopausal women had lost their uterus through surgical removal.[57] Four years later this figure was up to 35 percent.[37] By 1974 it was up even more—to 40 percent.[57] In 1975 hysterectomy had been performed on a startling 59 percent of the 369 menopausally distressed patients of one medical group.[10] More compelling is the recent study of 763 women whose menstrual history has been followed for the last forty-five years. These women were all healthy when they started recording their menstrual history; 31 percent had been hysterectomized before their menstrual cycles had stopped.[61] Figures are not yet available for that group to define how many will have had a hysterectomy throughout the full span of their lives. But by 1978, the lifetime chance for having a hysterectomy in the United States was estimated to be greater than 50 percent.[49] The incidence seemed to have stabilized at this level by 1983. Hysterectomy is second only to D & C or laparoscopy (examination of the interior of the abdomen) as the most common operation performed on women.[36] While this surgery may be justified, the reason for its increase has not been elucidated. We need to find out why.

Why?

Different reasons are given for the removal of the uterus. This is not surprising since different doctors have different attitudes about the importance of the uterus. Clearly, it should be removed when it is diseased and threatens your well-being.

Many gynecologists spoke out in 1976 at a medical meeting that was evaluating hysterectomy. One respected woman in particular listed, and we concur with her beliefs, the following reasons which are "appropriate indications for hysterectomy," given our current state of knowledge:

- premalignant states of localized invasive cancers of the cervix, endometrium, ovaries, or Fallopian tubes

- symptomatic nonmalignant conditions of the uterus such as leiomyomas (nonmalignant tumors of the uterine smooth muscle, also called fibroids) compressing adjacent pelvic structures, which gives rise to uterine bleeding—if the uterine bleeding is unresponsive to other nonsurgical treatments

- uterine bleeding that is not responsive to hormone therapy

- uterine pain or bleeding when hormone therapy would be dangerous

- diseased Fallopian tubes

- prolapse of the uterus due to loss of its supporting structure's health (if you had prolapse, the uterus would drop down into the vagina)
- cancer of adjacent structures
- uterine rupture[19]

There may be other important reasons for the surgery such as endometriosis, as any competent physician will advise. The important thing is for you to find unbiased, compassionate, expert advice. Before one removes a diseased organ, it is sensible to first try to heal it. The reason for excessive bleeding should first be determined and perhaps could be better treated with hormones (progesterone).[22]

How many of the hysterectomies being performed in the United States today are being done for one or more of the uncorrectable reasons listed above? We do not know.[7] There is no systematic and retrievable reporting system among the medical communities, except for the hospital record room and tissue committees, that would allow such information to be retrieved. These hospital committees are formed of medical professionals who accept the responsibility of reviewing the results of recent hospital activities, including the outcome of individual surgical operations. The information in the tissue committees is privileged in a legal sense and, therefore, not readily available.

From statements reported by gynecologists at medical meetings and in several published studies, it would appear that many hysterectomies are done for purposes of birth control (permanent sterilization), to prevent cancers, or "to improve the quality of life."[7, 18, 31] We believe that the removal of a healthy organ for reasons of birth control or cancer prevention is not in the best interest of the patient. Hysterectomy is major surgery and has its risks, both in pain and potential complications. There are, obviously, alternative methods of birth control that avoid hysterectomy. Before you undergo surgery, be sure that you have explored the other alternatives first. A complete review of alternatives to hysterectomy for birth control is available.[23] It is not wise for you to undergo major surgery unless you must. But if you must, it is important to know what to expect.

Types of hysterectomies and their aftereffects

There is confusion in regard to terminology. For most people a "hysterectomy" means the removal of the uterus, tubes, and ovaries and is often said to be a total hysterectomy. The correct names for the removal of uterus, tubes, and ovaries is a *total hysterectomy and bilateral salpingo ovariectomy.* If only the uterus and cervix are removed, this is correctly called a *total hysterectomy,* although in some colloquial expressions this removal of the uterus and cervix alone is called a partial hysterectomy because the tubes and ovaries remain. A *subtotal hysterectomy* is sometimes confused with a partial hysterectomy but is actually quite different. A subtotal hysterectomy means that the cervix is left behind. Figures 17, 18, and 19 depict the different kinds of hysterectomies.

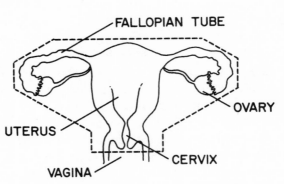

Figure 17 Total Hysterectomy and Bilateral Salpingo Ovariectomy

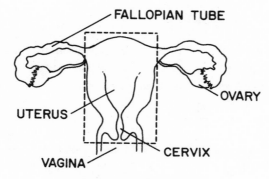

Figure 18　Total Hysterectomy

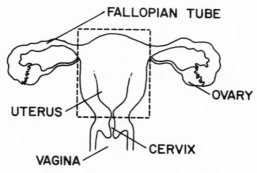

Figure 19　Subtotal Hysterectomy

The uterus can be removed in either of two ways: through the vagina or through a surgical opening in the abdominal wall. A good physician is in the best position to select the best approach for the particular case.

The vaginal hysterectomy is advisable when the anatomy allows for the easy removal of the uterus from below. For instance, in a woman who has borne many children the vaginal opening is generally more relaxed and permits this easy access. The second critical point necessary for allowing a vaginal hysterectomy is that the woman's individual health show no disturbances in either blood circulation or skeletal structure that might be aggravated by the prolonged operative position in stirrups that the body must assume. Finally, the surgeon should be proficient in this approach or be supervised by a skilled and experienced pelvic surgeon who is guiding and assisting him or her.

Both forms of the operation, vaginal and abdominal, produce about the same amount of sickness although the particular kinds of discomfort may vary.[19] Vaginal-hysterectomy patients may show a much higher incidence of postoperative fever and higher numbers of localized infections of the vagina. They also experience a greater postoperative vaginal blood loss.[66]

With both approaches, the intestine is sometimes inadvertently wounded. This is more likely to occur in patients with prior abdominal surgery. Depending on your medical history, you may have a greater or lesser risk of these operative complications. For example, if you have had a Caesarean delivery or pelvic inflammatory disease before the hysterectomy, you have a greater chance of having the intestines stuck onto the uterus or tubes or ovaries before the operation has begun. If this were your situation, your surgeon would first have to separate these tissues before he could proceed with the removal of the uterus. In the process of detaching these tissues, there is a chance that a wound to the intestine (caused by the separation itself) may lead to postoperative complaints. If this happens, the small bowel can become paralyzed, and until it heals a woman will have a good deal of digestive problems, principally vomiting and pain.[66]

Although the aftereffects of abdominal and vaginal hysterectomies are different, with either approach you might be sick afterward. After a hysterectomy most women (about 80 percent) have fevers, which most often come from either urinary-tract infections or from inflammation of pelvic tissue.[33] In other words, the aftereffects of a hysterectomy can be unpleasant.

Some studies present evidence that supports the theory that

the blood flow to the ovaries is temporarily altered when the uterus is removed.[29] As a result of this reduction in blood flow, the estrogen secretion (of young ovaries) or the other hormone secretions (of older ovaries) have been reported to be temporarily suspended.[58] There is an immediate hormone drop that is quite large. This has been observed to occur more often on the second day after surgery.[28] This reduction of the ovarian blood flow may account for the hot flashes that women often report right after hysterectomy. Commonly, the flashes reach their maximum by about the fourth or fifth day after surgery.[2] When the full blood flow is eventually restored, the flashes stop.

Not every surgeon's patients get flashes. One group of doctors reported that 69 percent of their patients experienced postoperative flashing;[51] another group rarely found flashing in women they interviewed after surgery.[12] What might explain the difference? Different surgical techniques may be the answer. Perhaps some techniques do not disrupt the flow of blood from the ovary. Other internal tissue traumas are common, including injury to the blood vessels in the operated pelvic area, the rectum, the bladder, and the ureters.[19, 32]

Bladder trouble is sometimes another problem of recovery from hysterectomy surgery.[21] The kinds of changes you can expect to experience include difficulty in voiding. This is related to the alterations in the sensation that are produced on separating the bladder from the uterus. In order to remove the uterus, the surgeon must separate these two organs, which are normally attached to each other. These urinary problems are always temporary, and some women do not experience them at all.

Sexual discomforts are also common. The temporary ones, such as pain on first attempting intercourse after surgery, indicate that coitus has been resumed too early. It is best to abstain from sexual intercourse until the healing is complete—that is, when you are no longer sore. After surgery the abdomen feels sore and is easily bruised. It commonly takes three to four months before coital pressure can be enjoyed rather than merely tolerated.[1] There is often a temporary narrowing and shrinking of the vagina. These various difficulties can combine to make sexual intercourse unpleasant at first. However, with a considerate and understanding partner, one who is willing to be gentle, resumption of coital activity can promote the return of pleasurable sex. Most women become sexually active again between two and four months after such surgery.[13]

There are also all sorts of complications that can occur after any surgery. Such a list is not included here. But most of the problems of hysterectomy surgery are annoying and not life-threatening. They are, however, sufficiently discomforting for you to seek a hysterectomy only if it is really necessary for you. Choose your surgeon carefully because these problems are less likely to happen with a highly skilled gynecological surgeon. There is a wide variation in the quality of surgeons, and finding a good one should be an important priority.

There may be occasions where differences of opinion are expressed concerning the need for hysterectomy. For example, a patient that has the desire for future procreation and has extensive fibroids of the uterus might better benefit from removal of these fibroid tumors (referred to as "multiple myomectomy") than from a hysterectomy since hysterectomy would preclude future childbearing. To save such a uterus may necessitate the seeking out of an experienced and able gynecological surgeon who is adept at such conservational surgery. The myomectomy may require a much longer operation than a hysterectomy because it can be technically more difficult and time-consuming for the surgeon to remove individual tumors and then repair the uterine areas from which they have been removed than to remove the entire uterus. If you are well informed, you should insist that your own special needs be reflected in the approach that the physician outlines for you. There is a delicate balance between the needs of the woman and the propriety of what the physician can and should do. There are no simple answers. Getting the proper opinion depends upon how you approach the specific physician and how you weigh the importance of what he or she and others offer to provide you with. The more knowledgeable you are, the better you are able to ask the right questions. We suggest that you look for satisfied patients as references.

You may want to find two surgeons who are not professionally connected with each other in order to allow you to get two independent opinions about the importance of surgery for your problem. To do this, each physician should form and render an opinion on the basis of personal judgment, and this should be a judgment that is unbiased by the knowledge of where and what judgment was rendered elsewhere. You will optimize objectivity if you require the same rigor of judgment about your case that researchers require of their studies. It is like the double-blind requirement, discussed earlier. If you lack tact, however, you could potentially be misunderstood and possibly find that you have insulted the person you are going to for help. While it is perfectly reasonable to seek two unbiased opinions, it is unreasonable to behave as though you do not trust the ability of your physician. You tread a delicate balance when you seek two truly objective opinions. If right from the start you are tactfully able to communicate the truth—that you are seeking two independent and unbiased judgments—you should be able to secure competent medical help. Yes, it will cost you an extra fee since some insurance companies may not reimburse for a second opinion. When you need the operation, it can enhance your well-being to have the surgery. In any event, it makes sense to consider carefully the reason for surgery before you decide to have your uterus removed.

Why keep your ovaries?

Some doctors routinely remove the ovaries when they remove the uterus. Current statistics indicate that for women over forty, half of those who undergo hysterectomy also have their ovaries removed.[18] Too commonly, one would hear comments like "As long as I'm cleaning out your uterus, I might as well clean out your ovaries too." With the development of modern science, reproductive researchers have provided clear evidence that shows how important your ovaries are no matter how old you are! Thus, the ovaries should not be removed unless they are diseased. Some gynecological surgeons—particularly the gynecologic oncologists —are beclouded by the great many ovarian cancers they see and tend to extrapolate the risk of cancer to retained ovaries. This occurs precisely because they are experts in that field and, therefore, tend to see a preponderance of malignant cases. Hence, such specialists may feel the need to remove ovaries in women routinely after age forty-five to fifty. We do not agree. We think that each case must be considered on its own merits. The actual studies suggest that ovarian cancer risk is not higher in those hysterectomized women who keep their ovaries compared to women who never had a hysterectomy. Moreover the removal does not assure the absolute prevention of ovarian tissue cancer.[60] These facts strongly suggest that ovariectomy of healthy ovaries is unnecessary.[3, 60] We predict that in the future women will have their ovaries monitored by ultrasound. Ultrasound permits an internal view of the body (like X-rays do) but does not bombard it with gamma radiation. Rather, it uses the echo characteristics of sound waves. These sound waves do not appear to be harmful.

Since the postmenopausal ovaries are active hormone producers (see Chapter 1 to review the facts), one can expect good benefits from retaining the ovaries. The removal of the ovaries will induce a profound shock and an immediate menopause. As described in Chapters 3 and 4, when the ovaries are removed from a premenopausal woman, one expects rapid skin aging,[26, 45] bone deterioration, and other hormone-related changes that would not occur if these hormone-producing glands (the ovaries) were retained. Even after age fifty, removal of the ovaries will cause physiological changes, and simply replacing estrogen and progestogen will not bring the hormonal environment back to its presurgical state.[56]

Since, as described in Chapter 1, a woman's ovaries probably continue to function throughout her life, it is not surprising that ovariectomy leads to loss of bone mass. Four years after ovariectomy, when no hormone replacement therapy is given, most young women show beginning signs of osteoporosis.[27] Even in the aging ovary, ovariectomy will influence the speed with which osteoporosis develops.

If you lose your ovaries before age fifty to fifty-five and don't take estrogens, your skin will begin aging rapidly. It will wrinkle, dry out, and sag much the way a plum turns into a prune. This condition will get worse as the time since the ovariectomy increases.[45] But there is hope. Hormone therapy seems to prevent this unfortunate condition.

Young women who are hysterectomized and retain their ovaries often continue to show a normal cycle of ovarian hormone secretion; and though menstruation has stopped, the other cyclic changes (like mood swings, breast swelling, etc.) often go on until the age of natural menopause.[4, 9, 16, 20, 47, 48] The postmenopausal ovary continues to produce hormones, and women in their sixties were shown to have active ovaries when tested during surgical procedures.[35]

During the menopause years it makes sense to retain the ovaries, if possible. Hysterectomy, both with and without ovariectomy, was evaluated in one study of 122,000 women. The women whose ovaries were retained enjoyed a reduced risk of heart attack (myocardial infarction) when compared with those women whose ovaries had been removed.[55] The younger the woman, the greater her benefit in keeping the ovaries intact; but at every age the ovaries provided a reduced risk of heart attack. Such a finding makes sense if you realize that, due to the estrogen (and possibly progesterone) secreted by the ovaries, women enjoy a lower heart-attack rate than men. In a different vein, it has recently been suggested that the "liberation" of women has produced a new breed of hard-driving women who, like their male counterparts, are going to be subject to an increased risk of heart disease because of coronary-prone behavior patterns.[64, 65] While such a suggestion may turn out to be true, it still seems likely that ovarian secretions will offer additional protection against heart disease, a protection that men do not enjoy. More on this hormonal influence is found in the section "Heart Disease" (pages 172–174) as well as in Appendix 2.

Remember that even when an older ovary stops producing estrogen, it continues to manufacture the androgens: androstenedione[39, 40] and testosterone.[40] If you are menopausal, losing your ovaries will result in a fall of androstenedione and testosterone in your blood levels. These hormones, along with estrogens, can be important to your health and sense of well-being. The ovaries continue to be vital organs even during menopause.[35, 38, 39, 40, 56, 59] Keep them if you can. Should your ovaries be routinely removed at hysterectomy? No! Is it safe to keep them in? Yes, it appears to be safe[46] unless uterine cancer is found or the ovaries are diseased—in which case your doctor will probably recommend that they be removed. But even the issue of cancer prevention by ovariectomy is controversial. Recent evidence has shown that ovariectomy of normal ovaries did not prevent cancer.[60] This makes routine ovariectomy less defensible.

What is the recovery period after hysterectomy like?

One California woman put it pretty clearly:

After my hysterectomy, I had the usual post operation discomfort. About one week after the surgery I became very depressed and cried all the time. My feelings reminded me of how I felt after I had child birth. I really had no reason for feeling so blue. My family and friends had been very supportive and loving. I had my tubes tied 7 years ago so it wasn't that I was upset about not being able to have children. I remember when I was taking a shower one day, I was crying so hard I thought I was drowning in my emotions. I talked to my doctor and he said it would pass. That probably there was a shock to my ovaries and that they had stopped producing estrogen and that it was a change in my chemistry that was causing my depression. He was right. In about a week later I felt much better. I have felt better all the time and the fact that I don't need to worry about heavy periods draining me every month is such a relief.

Things probably do settle down, but the recovery from the operation can, and often may, be difficult. Although some women seem to bounce right back after surgery, the vast majority find recovery a slow and painful process. One study compared 56 hysterectomized women with age-matched control women undergoing a variety of other surgical operations. Hysterectomy encompasses a more complicated abdominal surgery than most other operations. It is not surprising that it produces the slowest convalescence of all: on the average it took about 13 months for a woman to feel as if she were her old self, again and this compared with an average of 4.2 months for recovery from the other operations (e.g., removal of the appendix, thyroid, breast, gall bladder).[51]

Long-term problems and remedies

Sexual function deficits

The following are the most frequent difficulties that women encounter in resuming sexual activity after hysterectomy:

- dryness of the vagina and failure to lubricate during intercourse
- dyspareunia (painful intercourse)
- bleeding during intercourse
- loss of libido

Vaginal wetness in response to sexual arousal can occur with or without the uterus. But the cervix—the lower tip of the uterus —is responsible for a fluid that doubtless contributes moisture. In fact for cycling women, as their mid-cycle ovulatory stage approaches each month, this fluid becomes copious—more so than at any other time during the cycle. While physiologists may show that vaginal lubrication resulting from sexual arousal is unimpaired by hysterectomy and mainly originates in the vaginal walls, the total amount of fluid may be diminished by the loss of that produced by the cervix, particularly in younger women. For women past fifty-five, substantiation of a cervical contribution to vaginal moisture is not yet readily available.

The loss of libido

The loss of sexual desire after hysterectomy is common. This is true even when ovaries are retained.[17, 42, 62, 63] Between 25 percent and 45 percent of women lose their sexual appetite after losing their womb. Taking estrogens doesn't help.[63] In fact, one double-blind study showed that estrogen eliminated the dyspareunia but did not influence the libido.[17] These libido effects have been studied at different times and were found to occur at all times studied: immediately;[42] up to two years after surgery;[63] and even five years after the operations.[17]

Why would a decrease in sexual desire follow the loss of a uterus? First, the uterus itself could be a sexual center whose pleasure helps promote appetite. The studies at the University of Pennsylvania among young women and at Stanford University among women in menopausal transition support such an idea.[14] Others have considered it also.[42] Here is what one woman had to say:

The greatest change since the surgery is this. Before, each time the penis is pushed hard against the cervix, I would feel intense excitement deep inside me, huge waves of pleasure going from the area of the cervix all through my torso. This was by far the most exciting part of sex for me, the real climax. I've tried to be satisfied with the orgasms I get from stimulation of the clitoris, that is mildly pleasurable contractions in the muscles in the front part of the vagina. Maybe I'll get used to it in time, but it isn't nearly as good, and I feel sad.[69]

Second, the uterus might produce and/or respond to hormones that are related to sexual appetite. So little is yet known in this respect that we can do no more than speculate.

Third, there may be psychological reasons for a decrease in sexual appetite after hysterectomy. Many women consider sexual pleasure integrally linked with childbearing. Knowing that childbearing days are over may decrease sexual appetite for such women. Still others may be involved in deteriorating relationships and find it convenient to use the fact of the operation as the "reason" for loss of libido.

Depression

The word "hysterectomy" has an interesting history. It is derived from the Greek and the Latin. The Greeks called the womb "hystera." The Latin "hystericus," suggesting disturbances of the womb, became associated with the English word "hysteria," an emotional disorder. The thinking at that time implied that the uterus has a controlling influence on the female brain.

Depression hits in different ways at different times in life. There are occasions when being depressed is normal. To react to a serious loss with depression is to be expected. Hysterectomy produces a loss of something very important. Not surprisingly, younger women—those in their childbearing years—are more prone to depression after hysterectomy than older women.[41, 50] If you lose your ability to have children before you have had a chance to complete your family, you have reason to be depressed; and 55 percent of women under forty who have this surgery do go through a period of real and, by established medical standards, severe depression afterward.[50]

But sometimes depression is not to be "expected." A menopausal woman whose family is complete has no obvious reason to bemoan the loss of her womb. And, therefore, more troubling is a series of studies that have suggested a menopausal posthysterectomy depression syndrome. In 1957 a paper reported on a group of women who had been hysterectomized and followed for ten years by one physician. The author suggested that most postoperative troubles begin after the last routine follow-up that a surgeon performs. She showed how physicians could be under the false impression that women recover nicely from hysterectomies because, usually, the doctors have stopped seeing their patients by the time the troubles begin.[15] Here are the facts: in the first year after operation 83 percent were satisfied with the results of their surgery; between one and five years after the operation 41 percent were satisfied; between six and ten years postoperative this figure dropped down to 33 percent. Another investigator, eleven years later, found that there was a two-year delay after surgery before the postoperative depression was most likely to happen.[6]

Hysterectomy is more likely to produce depression than other operations. When hysterectomized women were compared with age-matched women having other surgical operations, the hysterectomized women fared badly: 70 percent of the women who had their uterus removed had a severe depression, which was more than double the rate of other postoperative depressions.[50] Two other published studies confirmed this finding.[6, 41]

Why is hysterectomy so much more terrible an operation than other surgical procedures? Or is it? Is it possible that women who are depressed are more likely to have their uterus taken out than women who are not depressed? Unfortunately, it looks as though this is true.[24, 44]

One investigator demonstrated that in large population samples, the highest incidence of depressive illness occurs in women who are going through their change of life. In that age span 40 percent of the women show scores indicative of real clinical depression.[5] This 40-percent figure compares with a lower (25 percent) figure for all other age groups in that study. Women in the forty-five- to forty-nine-year-old age group (the menopausal transition years) are most likely to develop depression.[5] Preoperative depression was measured in age-matched women before hysterectomy and before other surgical operations. And preoperative depression was twice as common in the women about to undergo hysterectomy.[51] Hysterectomy was most difficult when it occurred during the change of life and best tolerated in women over the age of fifty-five.[15]

Depressed patients frequently have perceptions that their symptoms are worse than they would have judged them to be if the patients were in a nondepressed state.[25] Since many women slated for hysterectomy appear to be scheduled on the basis of self-report of their heavy bleeding symptoms,[31] it is possible that the uterus is sometimes coming out because the patient is depressed. In fact one study showed that women who were depressed preoperatively were much more likely to have a normal uterus (discovered after the surgery) than women who were not depressed preoperatively.[6] Patients often do not appreciate that a hysterectomy may not correct the symptoms that produced a depression. What a terrible thought! Obviously, it doesn't happen in every case, but any case in which it does is unfortunate.

Time and the care of a loving person are probably the most reliable emollients for the depression that women feel after a hysterectomy.[34] Love is always available in the form of service to others in one context or another. If you suffer a depression, try helping someone less fortunate than you are. Maintain contact with other people. It usually helps, and, as an added bonus, you help another person. But if you find you are unable to overcome a debilitating depression, seek medical help. There are remedies available in the form of psychotherapies and drugs.

Heart disease

Hysterectomy results in an increased risk for heart disease, according to one investigator who reviewed many small studies. The conclusion reached was that the risk of coronary heart disease increases three- to fivefold over what is expected in similar-aged women who have their uterus intact.[11] A closer look at the individual studies indicates that while hysterectomy alone often shows negative heart health effects, ovariectomy plus hysterectomy may be even worse when no hormone therapy is taken. If you must give up your uterus, the retention of your ovaries may help limit the risk.

In one large-scale evaluation, compared to other women of the same age who had no surgery, ovariectomy was associated with three times the risk of heart disease (nonfatal myocardial infarction). The younger the woman, the greater the risk for having a heart attack. For example, a thirty-five-year-old woman who had an ovariectomy was more than seven times likely to have a heart attack than a thirty-five-year-old woman who did not have the surgery. Hysterectomy by itself, with the ovaries left intact, did not seem to be a risk factor in this study.[55] Apparently, the risk of heart attack increased in that sample only when the ovaries were also removed at hysterectomy. While a heart attack proves the presence of heart disease, the process that precedes the attack is often silent but insidious. Several studies have explored the question of whether hysterectomy increases the risk of developing heart disease. The evidence suggests that it may, although the issue is not yet fully resolved.

Atherosclerosis

Atherosclerosis, a condition in which the lining of the blood vessels becomes so clogged with cholesterol droplets that circulation is sometimes blocked, is a serious problem for many older people. Atherosclerosis leads to heart disease. Ovariectomy significantly increases the incidence of the problem when no estrogen replacement therapy is offered.[53, 68] In one study of several hundred hysterectomized women, those whose ovaries and uterus were removed before the age of forty-five showed four times the incidence of atherosclerosis than those whose ovaries were retained.[54] But a different team of investigators, asking similar questions, concluded that any hysterectomy (with or without ovariectomy) significantly increased the risks of atherosclerosis in younger and older women.[52] In the first study (claiming apparent similarity for risk of both surgeries) there was, however, a difference in cholesterol levels that appeared to relate to the presence or absence of ovaries in the body. Cholesterol levels were consistently higher among those hysterectomized women whose ovaries were removed than among those whose ovaries were retained. Levels increased with age, they increased even more for any given age when hysterectomy was performed, and they increased even further if ovariectomy was added to the hysterectomy.[52] *One may conclude that hysterectomy increases the rate of precipitators to heart disease and that ovariectomy compounds the problem.* Why the removal of the uterus, with the retention of the ovaries, should influence heart-disease rate is not known. Some investigators have suggested that the presence of the uterus may contribute something that keeps the ovaries more active,[52] but such a theory is only speculation. It needs to be tested by rigorous scientific research. Estrogens, in some as yet undiscovered way, appear to prevent the development of heart disease. For those who smoke, the risks of these surgeries may be worse since smoking greatly increases the chance for atherosclerotic disease. Reports have not yet been published to address directly this combination of factors to see if they compound the risks when occurring simultaneously.

Hormone replacement therapy after hysterectomy

The evidence looks compelling and good that HRT is beneficial. Two reports, one in 1975 and a follow-up in 1977, studied more than 1,000 women for up to seven years after their hysterectomies.[8, 9] All of these women were taking estrogen replacement therapy. If the ovaries were intact, the therapy began when menopausal symptoms (hot flashes, night sweats, etc.) began. If the ovaries were removed, estrogen therapy began immediately after the operation. The hormone doses were prescribed at the lowest level needed to maintain comfort. Results were clear in showing a marked drop in deaths from all causes. At every age the death and disease rates were much lower among estrogen users than in age-matched comparison populations who were not taking estrogens. The hormones improved the health outlook. The main improvement in longevity came because of reduced heart-attack rates and reduced cancer deaths. Both of these diseases, as described earlier, have certain connections with hormone levels. Nonhormone-related deaths (car accidents, for example) were equivalent in both the patient population and the population norms. Taking hormones, especially when there is no uterus to stimulate into a hyperplasia, appears to maximize one's health, longevity, and well-being. But to undergo hysterectomy in order to take hormones without risk doesn't make sense even though death after hysterectomy is unlikely.

One more point to know about is also important. You might

hear about the often-cited, very impressive Boston Collaborative Study which followed the cardiac health of a large population of men and women for many years. In this study fourteen of the postmenopausal women developed heart disease, and the authors noted that half of them used estrogen therapy and half did not. Although at first glance it seems as though the taking of hormones may be associated with heart disease,[30] a closer look does not support that conclusion. Nor do results of an earlier study that compared estrogen use to no estrogen use among 600 hysterectomized and oophorectomized women to test directly whether hormones were bad for hysterectomized women.[52] Hormone use did not increase the risk of heart disease in hysterectomized women, although the operation did increase the risk of heart disease over age-matched women who did not undergo hysterectomy. In the Boston Collaborative Study, of the fourteen postmenopausal women who developed heart disease, twelve had been hysterectomized at an age younger than their natural menopause. Information was not available that could tell how many of these twelve had also been ovariectomized. Since we know that hysterectomy and ovariectomy increases the risk of coronary heart disease, it may be that the precipitating factor in these cases of heart disease was related to the premenopausal hysterectomy, not to the hormone use. Unfortunately, we cannot test the question properly with the facts available. The data that were published in the Boston Study did not break down the facts that would be needed to properly analyze cause-and-effect relationships. One would need to know what dosages and durations of hormones had been taken, how much time had passed without any hormone therapy in these hysterectomized women, how many hysterectomized women were taking estrogen compared to a population of similar-aged nonhysterectomized women, and so forth. Adequate epidemiological studies are extremely difficult to design well. But from the large-scale studies of hysterectomized women taking estrogen replacement therapy, it seems clear that the overwhelming effect of HRT is beneficial to heart health in mature (over age fifty) women.

Summary

Although having a hysterectomy is a relatively safe operation, it is still serious surgery. We have listed the appropriate indications for hysterectomy. If your uterus is incurably diseased, having the operation can enhance your well-being. But be prepared. In addition to the pain of recovery, a postoperative bout of hot flashes is likely. There is also the chance of a decrease in libido and/or a change in your sexual response as well as a possible period of posthysterectomy depression.

9 / Conclusions

Trusting yourself

Some people live much longer than others largely because their bodies function better. The journey from full function to complete loss of function takes different routes in different individuals. Life-threatening diseases—the cancers, the loss of heart function or other blood-associated diseases like strokes, and diabetes —are the most common causes of death. Certain behaviors like smoking and highly stressful living clearly decrease the opportunity for healthy function.

Hormone replacement therapy has some very real benefits. When experienced with full knowledge and attendance to the various dangers (high-risk categories were listed in Chapter 6), it can enhance living tremendously. You may not need it. There appears to be a great individual variation in body changes throughout the life span, and these changes help determine who will benefit from hormone replacement therapy. There are some who say that hormone replacement therapy is "unnatural." But consider the following before deciding whether "natural" is necessarily better.

Scarcely over a hundred years ago women knew nothing of birth control. Married, sexually active women often became baby-making machines, reproducing constantly. They often died young of changes caused by physical and reproductive exhaustion. Birth-control measures (an "unnatural" process) increased the capacity of women to live free from such danger. Birth control also carries risks. But if we are wise, we use the benefits of biomedical innovation.

Your physician

Women may have various symptoms during the pre-, peri-, and postmenopausal phases of their lives. Different aspirations and perceptions of what is proper in life have a tremendous influence on how a woman's womb, ovaries, and hormone levels are viewed —not only by the woman but also by the physician. Not only is there a difference from one woman to the next, but there are differences in the same woman in the different stages of her life. These differences in perspective also apply to physicians, and even in the same physician from one phase of his or her training and experience to another phase of his or her professional life. It is, therefore, obvious that treatment can vary in accordance with maturity of judgment and knowledge. These variations in judgment will be reflected in the way you and your physician manage your health care. It is very important that he or she be kind, compassionate, and dedicated to your interests.

If you decide that hormones might help you, you will need to find a knowledgeable physician who can examine you, evaluate your medical history, and then discuss the options with you. Since your choice of a physician will radically affect the kind of treatment you can expect to receive, we recommend that you make real efforts to seek a doctor with whom you feel comfortable enough to ask questions and get understandable answers. Ask the people you know for recommendations, or try calling your county medical society or local hospital to start.

Once you have found a physician, your medical care will begin with a physical examination. Most likely, your doctor will check and record your weight and blood pressure, analyze a sample of your urine, examine your breasts, and perform a pelvic examination in which the vagina and cervix is evaluated. A blood test to check for the possibility of anemia as well as an evaluation of cholesterol levels may also be useful.

If you both decide on hormone therapy, a regular schedule for endometrial checkups will be planned. Usually, there is no need for endometrial assessment if you are going to take estrogen and at least ten days of progestin each month. But if you plan on taking only estrogen, your doctor will probably first want to check your endometrium and then follow this up by checking it every six months thereafter. The procedure for endometrial assessment was described in Chapter 6. An alternative to this endometrium examination (one that appears to be equally effective) is the use of the Progestin Challenge Test. This was described in Chapter 6 also. The challenge-test concept is new, so you would be wise to follow all information on this test that is sure to come out in the next few years.

In any event, you can maximize your health care by having written records of your personal history. It is easy to jot things down accurately when they are happening but surprisingly difficult to remember accurately once a few years have passed. Whenever you start recording your medical history, you set the stage (for you and for your daughters and granddaughters) for the detection of potential problems early enough to nip them in the bud. Annual health charts appear in the back of this book. They are intended as a personal diary for you to record what is happening. Please turn to page 243 for more information.

Appendix 1

The Studies on Hormone Replacement Therapy and Hot Flashes

The studies are absolutely consistent with each other in showing the relief that estrogen and opposed estrogen provides to women suffering from hot flashes.[5, 7, 10, 13] A few examples are detailed in this appendix.

One report[2] evaluated 369 patients with menopausal distress who were given "titrated" doses of estrogens (17β estradiol). In other words, if a particular hormone dose did not work, the dose was increased until it did. By using this method, excellent relief of symptoms was reported by 96 percent of the women studied with 76 percent of the women reporting that their hot flashes had totally disappeared. Total disappearance of sweating was reported by 80 percent of the women, of tingling by 91 percent, and of genital atrophy by 88 percent. Estriol, even in its lowest doses (2 mg. per day), was also usually effective at relieving menopausal flashes.[13] When the lowest doses of estriol failed to provide total relief, higher doses increased the beneficial response.

Double-blind studies that compare placebo to estrogen therapy have also been reported. One group compared the effects of Premarin (1.25 mg. per day taken three out of four weeks) to placebo (taken on the same schedule) on women who were experiencing severe menopausal distress.[3] Premarin was significantly more effective than placebo in relieving hot flashes, insomnia, irritability, anxiety, urinary frequency, general well-being deficits, and memory. There was no evidence that Premarin helped backache, joint aches, or libido. Interestingly, there was a highly significant placebo effect on problems of vaginal dryness, memory, urinary frequency reduction, and "youthful" skin appearance; but the placebo effect (on vaginal dryness, memory, etc.) was not as pronounced as the effect recorded when hormones were taken. We can conclude that some distress can be reduced by some process of faith in the treatment but that hormones work more reliably.

Double-blind studies that compared placebos, sedatives, and antihypertensive drugs to different brands of estrogen among women with menopausal hot flashes have also been published.[4, 5, 9, 11] They show that hormones are most effective, placebos are least effective, and the other drugs fall somewhere in between. For example, in one study among thirty women given placebos, 29 percent said things had improved although none reported disappearance of her flashes. Sedatives eliminated the flashes in 28 percent of a different group of fifty-six women. In contrast, between 68 percent and 92 percent of the women taking different regimens of hormone therapies found total relief from hot flashes. This seemed to be a function of which hormone was given. Even when total disappearance of symptoms failed to occur on estrogen therapy, every woman given these hormones noticed some improvement. Conjugated equine estrogen was the most effective agent tested in this study, but others were also helpful —estradiol valerianate and estriol in several different doses.[9]

Vaginal cream—both Estrace (.2 mg.) and Premarin (1.25 mg.)—as well as sublingual tablets (.5 mg. every other day) have all been tested and shown to be fully effective at relieving hot flashes.[12] Synthetic and natural estrogens eliminate hot flashes.[1, 8, 10] For twenty-two weeks in one study,[6] estrogen (100 mg.) implants, a form of hormone that is surgically inserted via a tiny incision, also were effective. Implants are less desirable because they require surgery, but they work as well as other forms of estrogen therapy.

The results are unambiguous. Estrogen therapy relieves hot flashes.

Appendix 2

The Studies on Cardiovascular Health and Hormones

A number of investigators have evaluated different aspects of heart disease with respect to hormone use. It is important to understand that while estrogen replacement therapy has been common for many years, progestin opposition to the estrogen therapy was not common. Because progestin has only recently become widely used, and studies to evaluate its effects require several years to complete, there is less information available on progestin than on estrogen in menopausal heart health. Moreover, biomedical investigators are only now working to determine the appropriate dose of progestin to prescribe. Therefore, it is critically important in evaluating the association between hormones and heart health to note the particular doses of particular hormone therapy regimens. For example, if a high dose of progestin were harmful, a low dose could be very helpful.

Viewed from this historical perspective—that estrogen treatment came first, then a lowering of estrogen doses, then the addition of progestin opposition, followed now by a new trend toward lowering the doses and increasing the number of days that progestins are taken each month—the studies discussed below will clarify an issue that has long appeared confusing because specific attention was not always paid to the details of dosage.

Hormones and blood pressure

Blood-pressure changes have been evaluated before, during, and after hormone replacement therapy regimens, and results suggest that for the vast majority of women there are no bad effects.[14] There are exceptions, however, and, if you do take hormones, it is important to have your blood-pressure levels checked regularly.

In one double-blind study comparing Premarin (1.25 mg.) to placebo, no elevation in either systolic or diastolic blood pressure was noted in association with hormone use. In fact there was a fall in the systolic blood pressure in both conditions.[6]

In another study, fifty women, forty-five to fifty-five years old, were placed on estrogen therapy (estradiol valerate) or placebo six months after having their ovaries removed. Blood pressure was measured before the treatment began, then three, six, and nine months later.[34] For forty-eight of the fifty patients there were no significant changes in diastolic blood pressure on any treatment. Two of the fifty patients were exceptions. They showed a marked elevation of diastolic blood pressure. In another study women taking estrogen, or estrogen opposed by progestin, were followed before, during, and after going off HRT, and these women were compared to a third group who took a placebo. Both systolic and diastolic blood-pressure levels were significantly lower during either hormone regimen, with a return to the higher pretreatment level after stopping the hormones. Placebo users did not show significant changes in diastolic pressure, although their systolic pressure did drop a little while taking placebo.[15] Diastolic pressure appears to be the most critical pressure measure in the risks that hypertension offer for heart disease, and diastolic pressure seems to be unimpaired by hormones.

Another group studied 570 women, all of whom had high blood pressure. Five of the 570 hypertensive patients had passed their menopause, and each of the five were also taking estrogens.[8] Each of these five menopausal women was taken off the estrogens, and the blood-pressure level of each returned to normal—taking from one to seven months to normalize. How shall we interpret these apparently conflicting studies? One should realize that only 1 percent of these hypertensive patients were menopausal. Since there were so few women to study (five), it would be foolish to draw any sweeping conclusions about all menopausal women from it—particularly in light of the studies that evaluate large groups of hormone users. One can say that if you develop high blood pressure on hormone therapy, then you should stop taking hormones and have your hypertension evaluated. If it persists or returns on HRT, then HRT is not for you. Notwithstanding the generally good picture, these exceptions lead us to suggest that women who take hormones should routinely have their blood pressures checked just to be sure that they are not the exceptions to the general rule of blood-pressure safety in response to hormone therapies.

Atherosclerosis and heart attack

Atherosclerosis (hardening of the arteries which predisposes a person to heart disease) does not appear to be increased by the use of hormone therapy. One prospective study of 1,900 women could find no association between the use of estrogen and the subsequent development of atherosclerotic heart disease.[16]

Possible relationships between hormone use and myocardial infarction (heart attack) have also been considered. For an eleven-year interval 15,500 women residents in a retirement community were evaluated.[23] Of these women, 220 suffered a heart attack for the first time in their lives. Analysis of the records showed that heart-attack victims were no more likely to have used hormone replacement therapy than the other age-matched women in the retirement community. Another retirement-community study reported similar conclusions.[28]

Myocardial infarction was also studied in detail by the Framingham Study (an ongoing prospective evaluation of a population in Massachussets). In respect to menopause and coronary heart disease, 2,873 Framingham women were followed up for twenty-four years. No premenopausal woman ever developed a myocardial infarction or died of coronary heart disease. Such events were more common among postmenopausal women over age forty-five, whether the menopause began naturally or resulted from hysterectomy.[10]

The Framingham investigators then looked at those women who took estrogens (but they did not describe the brand or dose) and compared these women to those who did not take estrogens to see if hormone use influenced the rates of death or the rates of heart attacks. Death rates were not affected by estrogen use. Just as the retirement community described earlier showed, about 7 percent of the postmenopausal women died from coronary heart disease, and this occurred whether or not hormones were used. Heart-attack rates also were not affected by the use of estrogens. A third evaluation of natural-estrogen use in postmenopausal women also showed that estrogens do not increase and may actually reduce the likelihood of heart attack. Among 7,000 healthy menopausal women studied, 5 percent were found to be users of HRT; among 336 menopausal patients who had suffered a heart attack, only half as many, 2.5 percent, used these menopausal hormones.[27] Duration of treatment and age of the women were equivalent in both groups.[27] This study suggests that estrogen may have some protective effect against heart attack.

There are probably exceptions to the general rule that hormones are not involved with increased risks of heart attacks at the menopause, and regular blood-pressure checkups might help serve to distinguish those in the risk category from those who can safely take hormones. The increased risk, for those at risk, is very small. If you are one whose blood pressure is higher than normal, you might consider not taking hormone therapy. If your blood pressure is normal when on hormone therapy, it appears that you will not be at risk of heart disease.[23]

Studies of coagulation factors in blood

The ability of your blood to coagulate properly is an essential health requirement. Studies have been conducted to test whether the relevant blood factors are impaired by estrogen or progestin use. Most laboratory studies reflect a less dynamic situation than exists in the body. Nonetheless, results show no impairment on natural estrogens,[15, 20] and at least one investigator has suggested that natural estrogens are the most sensible estrogens to use.[20]

In one study ten women who had been ovariectomized and later treated with estradiol valerate showed no significant changes in any of seventeen different coagulation factors during a one-month period of estrogen use.[29] In another report estriol succinate, in doses titrated to that minimum level necessary for relief of menopausal distress symptoms, was shown to have no significant effects on plasma coagulation factors in ten women who were followed for twelve months.[33] Apparently, natural estrogens do not alter blood coagulation factors. Progestin in combination with estrogen has also been tested and shows no dangerous effects on these blood coagulation factors either.[1]

Synthetic estrogens appear to be different from the natural ones. One investigator claimed that there were "profound risks" for those women who took ethinyl estradiol, a synthetic estrogen, and these risks persisted for nine months after hormone therapy stopped.[1] Other investigators also commented on these risks.[33] For a fuller discussion of synthetic hormone risks, see page 192, "Natural versus Synthetic Estrogens."

Serum cholesterol, lipid balance, and serum triglyceride studies

Women who have unusually high levels of the low-density lipoproteins in their blood have been identified as those who are most likely to have heart disease.[13] High-density lipoproteins, in direct contrast, have been shown to be beneficial to coronary health.[18] High-density lipoprotein is so named because the molecule (protein coupled to a kind of fat droplet called a lipid) has a higher proportion of protein than lipid. Apparently, when the lipid is balanced by relatively high protein concentration (i.e., high density), greater protection against clogged arteries occurs. Estrogens have been shown to increase the levels of these beneficial high-density lipoproteins.

Among 4,978 women, ranging from twenty-one to sixty-two years, at each age the average level of the high-density lipoprotein was higher in hormone users than among nonusers.[4] Young hormone users are usually taking birth-control pills. Older hormone users are generally taking estrogen replacement. Progestogens, when added to the estrogen, had the reverse effect, but it appears that this adverse progestogen influence on high density lipoprotein is limited to much higher doses of progestin than were recommended in Chapter 6.[11, 19, 24, 30]

Studies have shown that the fatter you get, the lower your high-density lipoprotein level will be.[4] So here lies another danger in being fat.

Menopausal women who take natural estrogens may enjoy the advantage of a higher level of these beneficial high-density lipoproteins than nonusers. Several studies of different natural estrogens showed this increase.[31, 35, 36] Synthetic estrogens also produced increases in these beneficial lipoproteins.[36]

Cholesterol levels (another predisposing factor for heart disease) have actually been shown to decline while menopausal women are on hormone therapy, thereby producing another beneficial effect.[2] And one group reported positive results after giving estrogen (estradiol valerate) to women to reduce their excessively high cholesterol levels. The treatment was effective.[31] Progestin opposition seems to facilitate this beneficial decline.[8, 11, 15]

Serum triglycerides (fats traveling in blood that also can cause heart disease) are increased in menopausal women who take synthetic estrogens, but they are not increased when menopausal women take natural estrogens.[15, 19, 36] Progestin effects depend on the dose. In one study using high doses of Norgestrel (1.8 mg. per day), progestins were shown to increase certain triglycerides.[31] Lower doses (levels corresponding to recommendations listed in Chapter 6) and other types have not been implicated as causing triglyceride increases.[15, 19, 31]

One estrogen that has been evaluated, (seminatural) estradiol valerate (2 mg. per day), produced no increases in blood cholesterol or triglycerides in one group of ten ovariectomized women being given hormone replacement.[29] Another study showed that neither estradiol (2 mg. per day) nor estriol (1 mg. per day) produced any significant changes in cholesterol or triglycerides when compared to placebo in one group of forty-nine postmenopausal women who were taking hormones for relief of menopausal distress.[37] Confirmation has been reported.[9] A third approach compared three natural estrogen brands—Premarin (high and low doses), Harmogen (a brand name for piperazine oestrone sulfate, packaged in Great Britain), and estradiol valerate—and evaluated three different serum (blood) lipids.[17] None of the hormones produced any significant changes in any of the serum lipids measured, and none of the lipids increased when progesterone was added. Another recent report has provided data that support these comforting findings.[7] Nonetheless, because the higher doses of progestins sometimes caused triglyceride and cholesterol changes,[11, 30] the newer lower doses may be more desirable.

Natural versus synthetic estrogens

In general, heart and blood health seems to be increased or unaffected by natural estrogens—as the studies just described have detailed. However, synthetic estrogens sometimes appear to have some dangerous side effects. In several reports[3, 19, 25, 26, 36] synthetic estrogens increased triglyceride levels while natural estrogens did not. A report evaluating responses to conjugated equine estrogen (natural) and ethinyl estradiol (synthetic) described significant rises in serum triglyceride levels on both low and high doses of ethinyl estradiol (20 or 50 micrograms per day) but no significant change on either of two natural estrogen doses (.625 or 1.25 mg. per day).[3] Here, seventeen ovariectomized women had been treated with each of four hormonal doses at different times. There is a growing appreciation of the possible risks of synthetic estrogen on menopausal heart health.[3, 14, 19, 20, 21, 24, 26, 27, 28, 32] Until these questions are fully resolved, we prefer natural estrogens.

Estrogens in young women

Young women appear to be physiologically different from mature postmenopausal women. It is important to realize that although in some cases estrogens (as oral contraceptives) have been associated with increased risks of various heart-disease factors, natural estrogens among older women have not been related to these risks. One unresolved area concerns the young woman who is hysterectomized and then wants to know whether estrogen therapy will do for her what it does for other menopausal women or whether it will work on her body as the oral contraceptives do on other young women.

Hysterectomy and hormones

Young women who become menopausal have an increased risk of heart disease. This appears to be true for those who do as well as those who do not take hormone replacement therapy, although since there are so few detailed studies on this the evidence is inconclusive. If you are under age forty-eight and have become menopausal by virtue of a hysterectomy (regardless of whether your ovaries were removed), it will be very important for you to monitor your cardiovascular health. It will also be wise for you to exercise regularly, stay slim, and follow a sensible diet. The large-scale studies of thousands of hysterectomized women on hormone replacement therapy showed no increased risk of heart disease.[5, 22] One small study that looked at women with heart disease who were taking hormone replacement therapy found that in almost all the cases the women were under forty-eight years old and had been hysterectomized.[12] This probably means that hysterectomy at a premenopausal age, not the hormones that were given in compensation, increased the risk of heart disease. But because of this study, we recommend that young hysterectomized women who take HRT schedule regular checkups of their cardiovascular health.

If you are older than forty-eight, the best evidence to date suggests that even if hysterectomized, you are not at any increased risk of death from heart disease if you take hormones than if you don't take hormones. Still, you would be wise to have your blood pressure and low-density lipoprotein levels monitored as a precaution. Blood pressure is easy to monitor. The low-density lipoprotein analysis requires that your health-care specialist remove a bit of blood for analysis in the laboratory. If either of these two measures shows you are above normal, then you will have to balance your decision about future hormone use by comparing the risks and benefits that your unique situation demands.

Appendix 3

The Calcium Values of Common Food Sources

TABLE I

Calcium Rich Foods

FOOD	PORTION	CALORIES	mg CALCIUM
Breads & Cereals			
Cream of Wheat, Instant	1 cup, cooked	130	185
Pabulum Cereal			
Barley or Rice	3/4 cup, cooked	108	188
Oatmeal or Mixed	3/4 cup, cooked	110	188
Thomas Protein Bread	1 slice	45	78
Dairy Products			
Cheese			
American	1 oz.	107	195
Cheddar	1 oz.	112	211
Cottage, Creamed	1 cup	239	211
Edam	1 oz.	87	225
Swiss	1 oz.	104	259
Ice Cream (Chocolate)	1/6 quart	174	131
Ice Milk (Vanilla)	1/6 quart	136	189
Milk			
Buttermilk, from Skim	1 cup	88	296
Skim	1 cup	89	303
Whole, Fat 3.5%	1 cup	159	288
Vanilla Pudding	1/2 cup	139	146
Yogurt from Skim with			
Nonfat Milk Solids	1 cup	127	452
Goat Milk	1 cup	163	315
Eggs			
Scrambled, Milk & Fat	1 medium	112	52

TABLE I *(continued)*

FOOD	PORTION	CALORIES	mg CALCIUM
Fish & Shellfish			
Flounder	3 oz.	61	55
Mackerel, Canned	3 1/2 oz.	192	194
Oysters, Raw	5–8 medium	66	94
Sardines, Canned	8 medium	311	354
Scallops, Cooked	3 1/2 oz.	112	115
Shrimp, Raw	3 1/2 oz.	91	63
Fruits & Seeds			
Figs, Dried	5 medium	274	126
Orange	1 medium	73	62
Sunflower Seeds	3 1/2 oz.	560	120
Syrups & Sweets			
Blackstrap Molasses	1 tbsp.	43	116
Maple Sugar	4 pieces (2 x 1 x 1/2 in.)	348	180
Chocolate Candy	1 bar (2 oz.)	296	52
Vegetables			
Artichoke	edible portion (base and soft end of leaves)	44	51
Beans			
Lima, Green, Cooked	6 tbsp.	111	47
Snap, Green, Cooked	1 cup	31	62
Wax, Yellow, Cooked	1 cup	22	50
Beet Greens, Cooked	1/2 cup	18	99
Broccoli			
Raw	1 stalk (5 in. long)	32	103
Cooked	2/3 cup	26	88
Cabbage, Savoy, Raw	2 cups shredded	24	67
Chard, Cooked	3/5 cup	18	73
Chicory	30 – 40 inner leaves	20	86
Collards, Cooked	1/2 cup	29	152
Endive	20 long leaves	20	81
Escarole	4 large leaves	20	81
Fennel, Raw	3 1/2 oz.	28	100
Leeks	3 – 4 (5 in. long)	52	52
Lettuce, Romaine	3 1/2 oz.	18	68
Mustard Greens, Cooked	1/2 cup	23	138
Parsley, Raw	3 1/2 oz.	44	203
Parsnips, Raw	1/2 large	76	50
Rutabagas, Cooked	1/2 cup	35	59
Spinach, Raw	3 1/2 oz.	26	93
Cooked	1/2 cup	21	83
Sweetpotatoes, Baked	1 large	254	72
Watercress, Raw	3 1/2 oz.	19	151

Source: Bowes and Church, *Food Values of Portions Commonly Used* (Philadelphia: Lippincott, 1970, 1980).

Acknowledgments

We wish to thank the many women and men whose interest and cooperation at various stages of the research for the book enabled us to write it. In the spring of 1979 Minnie Berg, Evelyn Cutler, and Jean Cutler obtained from 25 women anonymous information about personal details of their menopause. The following fall and spring in California another 300 women, as part of the Stanford Menopause Study, shared their personal experiences. Some came quite a distance to participate: from 30 miles north of San Francisco to 40 miles south of Santa Cruz. To all of you, our thanks.

Three Stanford students—Celeste Wiser, Emily Woo, and Caryn Truppman—are thanked for working so closely with Dr. Cutler in assembling data and readings on the menopause. She is grateful to the following women for having been research assistants: Pat Brick, Nancy Chilton, Diane Cohen, Patricia Congdon, Helen Hill, Barbara Hogue, Elizabeth Hunt, Jacqueline Hyde, Betty Land, Muriel Maverick, Ruth Miles, Barbara Morton, Joan Morton, Ida Murray, Rita Olson, Joan Piccard, Verne Rice, Sonya Urban, and Catherine Whalen.

The authors thank the scholars, scientists, and physicians who so generously shared their knowledge and expressed their perspectives—at Stanford: Dr. Julian Davidson, Dr. Seymour Levine, Dr. Emmet Lamb, Dr. Norma McCoy, Dr. George Feigen, Dr. Fredi Kronenberg, and Dr. Pat Cross; at the University of Kansas: Dr. Gilbert Greenwald; at the Medical College of Georgia: Dr. R. Don Gambrell; at the University of Pennsylvania: Dr. Santo Nicosia, Dr. David Goodman, Dr. Luis Blasco, Dr. Pedro Beauchamp, and Ms. Karen Mueller; at Abington Memorial Hospital: Dr. David Reese; at Beaver College: Dr. Richard Polis; and at the Monell Chemical Senses Center: Dr. George Preti.

To the individuals who were kind enough to read various versions and sections of the manuscript and note their critiques we are especially grateful: Dr. Melvin Moore, Sandy Brennan, Tricia and Bruce Weekly, Kathryn Burkhart, Adolph Berg, Dr. Norman Johnston, Dr. Arnold Jerrall, Ann Williams, Sara Bogdanoff, Joanne Hirsh, Martha Mockbee, Dr. Terry Allen, Karen Mayer, Janis Tyler Johnson, Adele Hertz-Gray, Selma Fiel, Helene Cohan, Teresa O'Dowd, and Lisa Biello.

To Scott Grossman, Stanley Fox, and Dr. Erika Friedmann for assistance in retrieving relevant studies, Dr. Cutler expresses her appreciation.

We thank the librarians at Beaver College, particularly Marion Green and Joe Charles, and at the Hospital of the University of Pennsylvania, Michael Rissinger, for their inexhaustible good cheer and help in retrieving numerous scientific papers.

Dr. Cutler would particularly like to thank Stephen Cutler for his continuing useful comments, his encouragement to journey to Stanford, his never-ending moral support, and especially his role in the purchase of a computer to enable efficient retrieval of the enormous amount of information to be assembled.

The authors are especially indebted to Dr. Julian Davidson for having provided the forum for beginning the study of menopausal women. It has been especially challenging for Dr. Cutler to work with him.

We particularly appreciate the people at W. W. Norton & Company. A consistently high level of professionalism characterizes this publishing company. Mary Cunnane, our editor, was both a pleasure to work with and a significant contributor to the clarity of the text. By her meticulous competence, Carol Flechner, our copy editor, has further enhanced the work.

The authors join each other in expressing pleasure and gratification for the opportunity of working together to create this book. Dr. Cutler formulated the idea of writing it through discussions with Dr. García while she was at Stanford. His willingness to continue to guide her studies as he had been doing since 1974 when she approached him as a graduate student in biology encouraged her to undertake the project. His patience and good will, combined with his extraordinary scientific competence, clinical expertise, and medical compassion, have been a continuing inspiration to her.

To Dr. David Edwards, Winnifred Cutler is also very grateful. In addition to his major contributions to the sections on sexuality, all his editorial work, which took many, many hours, is appreciated more than he can ever know. The authors are especially pleased to have remained on cordial terms with each other on the completion of the numerous revisions which produced the final copy.

This very complex subject of menopausal physiology and psychology has offered a fascinating journey for the three of us.

Bibliography

Reference citations in the biomedical sciences follow a commonly accepted, abbreviated format. Should you wish to locate any citation and be unfamiliar with the notation form used, the reference librarian will be able to direct you. The abbreviations used are listed below.

Acta Endocrinol *(Acta Endocrinologica)*
Acta Obstet et Gynecol Scand or **Acta Obstet Scand** *(Acta Obstetricia et Gynecologica Scandinavica)*
Am J Clin Nutr *(American Journal of Clinical Nutrition)*
Am J Epidemiol *(American Journal of Epidemiology)*
Am J Med *(American Journal of Medicine)*
Am J Clin Pathol *(American Journal of Clinical Pathology)*
Am J Obstet Gynecol *(American Journal of Obstetrics and Gynecology)*
Am J Psychiat *(American Journal of Psychiatry)*
Am J Roentgenology *(American Journal of Roentgenology)*
Ann Chir Gynaecol *(Annales Chirurgiae et Gynaecologiae [Helsinki])*
Ann Clin Res *(Annals of Clinical Research)*
Ann Int Med *(Annals of Internal Medicine)*
Ann NY Academy of Sciences *(Annals of the New York Academy of Sciences)*

Ann Surg   *(Annals of Surgery)*
Arch Intern Med   *(Archives of Internal Medicine)*
Arch Sex Beh   *(Archives of Sexual Behavior)*
Aust N Z J Med   *(Australian and New Zealand Journal of Medicine)*
Aust N Z J Obstet Gynaecol   *(Australian and New Zealand Journal of Obstetrics and Gynaecology)*
Br J Derm   *(British Journal of Dermatology)*
Br J Obstet Gynaecol   *(British Journal of Obstetrics and Gynaecology)*
Br J Prev Soc Med   *(British Journal of Preventative and Social Medicine)*
Br J Urol   *(British Journal of Urology)*
Brit Med J   *(British Medical Journal)*
Calif Tiss Res   *(Calcified Tissue Research [Berlin])*
Clin Endocrinol or **Clin Endocrinol [Oxf]**   *(Clinical Endocrinology [Oxford])*
Clin Endocrinol Metab   *(Clinics in Endocrinology and Metabolism)*
Clinics in Obstet & Gynaecol   *(Clinics in Obstetrics and Gynaecology)*
Clin Orthop or **Clin Orthop and Rel Res**   *(Clinical Orthopaedics and Related Research)*
Curr Med Res Opin   *(Current Medical Research and Opinion)*
Endocrinol   *(Endocrinology)*
Fertil Steril   *(Fertility and Sterility)*
Front Horm Res   *(Frontiers in Hormone Research)*
Geront Clin   *(Gerontologica Clinica)*
Gynec Invest   *(Gynecological Investigation)*
Gynecol Oncol   *(Gynecologic Oncology)*
I J Fertil   *(International Journal of Fertility)*
Int Arch Allergy Appl Immunol   *(International Archives of Allergy and Applied Immunology)*
Int J Health Services   *(International Journal of Health Services)*
Int J Cancer   *(International Journal of Cancer)*
Int J Obstet Gyn   *(International Journal of Obstetrics and Gynecology)*
Invest and Cell Path   *(Investigative and Cell Pathology)*
Israel J Med Sci   *(Israel Journal of Medical Sciences)*
JAMA   *(Journal of the American Medical Association)*
J Am Geriatr Soc   *(Journal of the American Geriatrics Society)*
J Am Pharm Assoc   *(Journal of the American Pharmaceutical Association)*
J Appl Physiol   *(Journal of Applied Physiology)*
J Biosoc Sci   *(Journal of Biosocial Science)*

J Bone Joint Surg (AM) *(Journal of Bone and Joint Surgery [American])*
J Chron Dis *(Journal of Chronic Diseases)*
J Clin Endocrinol Metab *(Journal of Clinical Endocrinology and Metabolism)*
J Clin Invest *(Journal of Clinical Investigation)*
J Endoc *(Journal of Endocrinology)*
J Geriatr Psychiatry *(Journal of Geriatric Psychiatry)*
J Kentucky Med Assn *(Journal of the Kentucky Medical Association)*
J Lab Clin Med *(Journal of Laboratory and Clinical Medicine)*
J Ob Gyn of the Br Commonwealth *(Journal of Obstetrics and Gynaecology of the British Commonwealth)*
J Physiol (Lond) *(Journal of Physiology [London])*
J Reprod Med *(Journal of Reproductive Medicine)*
J Sex Res *(Journal of Sex Research)*
J Steroid Biochem *(Journal of Steroid Biochemistry)*
J Toxicol Environ Health *(Journal of Toxicology and Environmental Health)*
Life Sci *(Life Sciences)*
Med J Aust *(Medical Journal of Australia)*
Med Sci Sports and Exercise *(Medicine and Science in Sports and Exercise)*
Med Times *(Medical Times)*
Metab Bone Dis & Rel Res *(Metabolic Bone Disease and Related Research)*
NEJM *(New England Journal of Medicine)*
NY State J Med *(New York State Journal of Medicine)*
Ob/Gyn News *(Ob.Gyn. News)*
Obstet Gynecol *(Obstetrics and Gynecology)*
Obstet Gynecol Surv *(Obstetrical and Gynecological Survey)*
Postgrad Med *(Postgraduate Medicine)*
Postgrad Med J *(Postgraduate Medical Journal)*
Proc Royal Soc of Med *(Proceedings of the Royal Society of Medicine)*
Royal Soc of Health J *(Royal Society of Health Journal)*
S Afr Med J or *S A Med J* *(South African Medical Journal)*
Scott Med J *(Scottish Medical Journal)*
Soc Biol *(Social Biology)*
Soc Sci Med *(Social Science and Medicine)*
Surg Gynecol Obstet *(Surgery, Gynecology and Obstetrics)*
Tex Med *(Texas Medicine)*

Chapter 1   The Sex Hormones

1. Abraham, G. E.; Lobotsky, J.; and Lloyd, W. 1969. Metabolism of testosterone and androstenedione in normal and ovariectomized women. *J Clin Invest* 48:696–703.
2. Barret, I.; Cullis, W.; Fairfield, L.; Nicholson, R.; MacNaughton, M.; Williamson, C. F.; and Sanderson, A. E. 1933. Investigation of menopause in 1000 women. Subcommittee of the Council of Medical Women's Federation of England. *Lancet* 106–8.
3. Bengtsson, C., and Lindquist, O. 1977. Coronary heart disease during the menopause. *Clinics in Obstet & Gynecol* 4:234–42.
4. Crilly, R. G.; Marshall, D. H.; and Nordin, E. E. 1979. Effect of age on plasma androstenedione concentration in oophorectomized women. *Clin Endocrinol* 10: 199–201.
5. Edman, C. D., and MacDonald, P. C. 1978. Effect of obesity on conversion of plasma androstenedione to estrone in ovulatory and anovulatory young women. *Am J Obstet Gynecol* 130:456–61.
6. Frumar, A.; Meldrum, D.; Geola, F.; Shamonki, I.; Tataryn, I.; Deftos, L.; and Judd, H. 1980. Relationship of fasting urinary calcium to circulating estrogen and body weight in postmenopausal women. *J Clin Endocrinol Metab* 50:70–75.
7. Grodin, J. M.; Siiteri, P. K.; and MacDonhald, P. D. 1973. Source of estrogen production in postmenopausal women. *J Clin Endocrinol Metab* 36:207.
8. Jick, H.; Porter, J.; and Morrison, A. D. 1977. Relation between smoking and age of natural menopause: report from the Boston Collaborative Drug Surveillance Program, Boston University Medical Center. *Lancet* 1:1354–55.
9. Judd, H. G.; Judd, G. E.; Lucas, W. E.; and Yen, S. S. C. 1974. Endocrine function of the postmenopausal ovary: concentration of androgens and estrogens in ovarian and peripheral vein blood. *J Clin Endocrinol Metab* 39:1020.
10. Judd, H. L.; Davidson, B. J.; Frumar, A. M.; Shamonki, I. M.; Lagasse, L. D.; and Ballon, S. C. 1980. Serum androgens and estrogens in postmenopausal women with and without endometrial cancer. *Am J Obstet Gynecol* 136:859–71.
11. Korenman, S. G.; Sherman, B. M.; and Korenman, J. C. 1978. Reproductive hormone function: the perimenopausal period and beyond. *Clin Endocrinol Metab* 7:625–43.
12. Longcope, C.; Hunter, R.; and Franz, C. 1980. Steroid secretion in the postmenopausal ovary. *Am J Obstet Gynecol* 138:564–68.
13. McNatty, K. P.; Makris, A.; DeGrazia, C.; Osathanondh, R.; and Ryan, K. J. 1979. The production of progesterone, androgens and estrogens by granulosa cells, thecal tissue and stromal tissue by human ovaries in vitro. *J Clin Endocrinol Metab* 49: 687–99.
14. Monroe, S. E., and Menon, K. M. J. 1977. Changes in reproductive hormone secretion during the climacteric and postmenopausal periods. *Clin in Obstet & Gynecol* 20:113–22.
15. Reyes, F. I.; Winter, J. S.; and Faiman, C. 1977. Pituitary-ovarian relationships preceding the menopause. I: A cross-sectional study of serum follicle-stimulating

hormone, prolactin, estradiol and progesterone levels. *Am J Obstet Gynecol* 129: 557–64.

16. Sherman B. M., and Korenman, S. G. 1975. Hormonal characteristics of the human menstrual cycle throughout reproductive life. *J Clin Invest* 55:699–704.
17. Treloar, A. E.; Boynton, R. E.; and Cowan, D. W. 1974. Menarche, menopause and intervening fecundability. *Human Biology* 16:89–107.
18. Vermeulen, A. 1976. The hormonal activity of the postmenopausal ovary. *J Clin Endocrinol Metab* 42:247–53.
19. Vermeulen, A. 1980. Sex hormone status of the postmenopausal woman. *Maturitas* 2:81–89.
20. Vermeulen, A., and Verdonick, L. 1978. Sex hormone concentration in post-menopausal women: relation to obesity, fat mass, age, and years post-menopause. *Clin Endocrinol* 9:59–66.
21. Wyshak, G. 1978. Menopause in mothers of multiple births and mothers of singletons only. *Soc Biol* 25:52–61.

ADDITIONAL RECOMMENDED READINGS

Abraham, G. E. 1974. Ovarian and adrenal contribution to peripheral androgens during the menstrual cycle. *J Clin Endocrinol Metab* 39:340–46.
Abraham, G. E.; Odell, W. D.; Swerdloff, R. S.; and Hopper, K. 1972. Simultaneous radioimmunoassay of plasma FSH, LH, progesterone, 17 hydroxyprogesterone and estradiol 17β during the menstrual cycle. *J Clin Endocrinol Metab* 34:312–18.
Adashi, E. Y.; Rakoff, J.; Divers, W.; Fishman, J.; and Yen, S. S. C. 1979. The effect of acutely administered 2 hydroxyestorone on the release of gonadotropins and prolactin before and after estrogen priming in hypogonadal women. *Life Sci* 25:20–51.
Anderson, D. C. 1976. The role of sex hormone binding globulin in health and disease. In *The endocrine function of the human ovary*, ed. V. H. T. James, M. Serio, and G. Giusti, pp. 141–58. London: Academic Press.
Balog, J. 1980. Obesity and estrogen. *Am J Obstet Gynecol* 138:242.
Calanog, A.; Sall, S.; Gordon, G.; and Southern, A. 1977. Androstenedione metabolism in patients with endometrial cancer. *Am J Obstet Gynecol* 129:553–56.
Carlstrom, K.; Damber, M.; Furuhjelm, M.; Joelsson, I.; Lunell, N.; and Von Schoultz, B. 1979. Serum levels of total dehydroepiandorosterone and total estrone in post-menopausal women with special regard to carcinoma of the uterine corpus. *Acta Obstet et Gynecol Scand* 58:179–81.
Chakravarti, S.; Collins, W. P.; Forecast, J.; Newton, J.; Oram, D. H.; and Studd, J. W. 1976. Hormonal profiles after the menopause. *Br Med J* 2:784–86.
Dor, P.; Muquardt, C. L.; Hermite, M.; and Borkowski, A. 1978. Influence of corticotrophin and prolactin on the steroid sex hormones and their precursors. *J Endoc* 77:263–64.
Flickinger, G. L.; Elsner, C.; Illingworth, D. V.; Muechler, E. K.; and Mikhail, G. 1977.

Estrogen and progesterone receptors in the female genital tract of humans and monkeys. *Ann NY Academy of Sciences* 286:180–89.

Grattarola, R.; Secreto, G.; and Recchione, C. 1975. Correlation between urinary testosterone or estrogen excretion levels and interstitial cell stimulation hormone concentrations in normal postmenopausal women. *Am J Obstet Gynecol* 121:380–81.

Gurpide, E. 1978. Enzymatic modulation of hormonal action at the target tissue. *J Toxicol Environ Health* 4:249.

Hutton, J. D.; Jacobs, H. S.; James, V. H. T.; Murray, M. A. D.; and Rippon, A. E. 1977. Episodic secretion of steroid hormones in post menopausal women. *J Endocr* 73:25P.

Jacobs, H. S.; Hutton, J. D.; Murray, M. A. D.; and James, V. H. T. 1977. Plasma hormone profiles in postmenopausal women before and during oestrogen therapy. *Br J Obstet Gynaecol* 84:314.

Judd, H. L., and Yen, S. S. C. 1973. Serum androstenedione and testosterone levels during the menstrual cycle. *J Clin Endocrinol Metab* 36:475–81.

Judd, S. J.; Rakoff, J. S.; and Yen, S. S. C. 1978. Inhibition of gonadotropin and prolactin release by dopamine: effect of endogenous estradiol levels. *J Clin Endocrinol Metab* 47:494–98.

Kwa, H. G.; Bulbrook, R. D.; Cleton, F.; Verstraeten, A. A.; Hayward, J. L.; and Wang, D. Y. 1978. An abnormal early evening peak of plasma prolactin in nulliparous and obese postmenopausal women. *Int J Cancer* 22:691–93.

Larsson-Cohn, U.; Johansson, E. D.; Kagedal, B.; and Wallentin, L. 1977. Serum FSH, LH and oestrone levels in postmenopausal patients on oestrogen therapy. *Br J Obstet Gynaecol* 85:367–72.

Longcope, C. 1971. Metabolic clearance and blood production rates of estrogens in postmenopausal women. *Am J Obstet Gynecol* 111:778–81.

Longcope, C.; Pratt, J. H.; Schneider, S. H.; and Fineberg, S. E. 1978. Aromatization of androgens by muscle and adipose tissues in vivo. *J Clin Endocrinol Metab* 46:146–52.

MacDonald, P. C.; Edman, C. D.; Hemsell, D. L.; Porter, J. C.; and Siiteri, P. K. 1978. Effect of obesity on conversion of plasma androstenedione to estrone in postmenopausal women with and without endometrial cancer. *Am J Obstet Gynecol* 130:448–55.

Medina, M.; Scaglia, H. E.; Vazquez, G.; Alatorre, S.; and Perez-Palacios, G. 1976. Rapid oscillation of circulating gonadotropins. *J Clin Endocrinol Metab* 43:1015–19.

Milewich, L.; Gomez-Sanchez, C.; Madden, J. D.; Bradfield, D. J.; Parker, P. M.; Smith, S. L.; Carr, B. R.; Edmanb, C. H.; and MacDonald, P. C. 1978. Dehydroisoandrosterone sulfate in peripheral blood of premenopausal, pregnant, and postmenopausal women and men. *J Steroid Biochem* 9:1159–64.

O'Dea, J. P.; Wieland, R. G.; Hallberg, M. C.; Lerena, L. A.; Zorn, E. M.; and Genuth, S. M. 1979. Effect of dietary weight loss on sex steroid binding, sex steroids and gonadotropins in obese postmenopausal women. *J Lab Clin Med* 93:1007–8.

Poliak, A.; Seegar-Jones, G.; and Goldberg, I. V. 1968. Effect of human chorionic gonadotropin on postmenopausal women. *Am J Obstet Gynecol* 101:731–39.

Rader, M. D.; Flickinger, G. L.; de Villa, G. O.; Mikuta, J. J.; and Mikhail, G. 1973. Plasma estrogen in postmenopausal women. *Am J Obstet Gynecol* 116:1069–73.

Sherman, B. M.; West, J. H.; and Korenman, S. G. 1976. The menopausal transition: analysis of LH, FSH, estradiol, and progesterone concentrations during menstrual cycles of older women. *J Clin Endocrinol Metab* 42:629–36.

Taylor, M. A.; Chapman, C.; and Hayter, C. J. 1977. The effect of altering thyroid hormone concentrations on plasma gonadotropins in postmenopausal women. *Br J Obstet Gynaecol* 84:254–57.

Wise, A. J.; Gross, M. A.; and Schalch, D. A. 1973. Quantitative relationship of the pituitary gonadal axis in post-menopausal women. *J Lab Clin Med* 81:28–36.

Chapter 2   The Change of Life

1. Ballinger, C. B. 1975. Psychiatric morbidity and the menopause: screening of general population sample. *Br Med J* 3:344–46.
2. Barret, I.; Cullis, W.; Fairfield, L.; Nicholson, R.; MacNaughton, M.; Williamson, C. F.; and Sanderson, A. E. 1933. Investigation of menopause in 1000 women. Subcommittee of the Council of Medical Women's Federation of England. *Lancet* 106–8.
3. Bart, P. 1971. Depression in middle aged women. In *Women in a sexist society*, ed. V. Gornick and B. K. Moran. New York: Mentor.
4. Bye, P. G. 1978. Review of the status of oestrogen replacement therapy. *Postgrad Med J* 54:7–10.
5. Campbell, S., and Whitehead, M. 1977. Oestrogen therapy and the menopausal syndrome. *Clinics in Obstet & Gynecol* 4:31–47.
6. Casper, R. F., and Yen, S. S. C. 1981. Menopausal flushes: effect of pituitary gonadotropin desensitization by a potent luteinizing hormone releasing factor agonist. *J Clin Endocrinol Metab* 53:1056–58.
7. Casper, R. F.; Yen, S. S. C.; and Wilkes, N. M. 1979. Menopausal flushes: a neuroendocrine link with pulsatile luteinizing hormone secretion. *Science* 205:823–25.
8. Chakravarti, S.; Collins, W. P.; Thom, M. H.; and Studd, J. W. 1979. Relations between plasma hormone profiles, symptoms and response to oestrogen treatment in women approaching the menopause. *Br Med J* 1:983–85.
9. Coope, J.; Williams, S.; and Patterson, J. S. 1978. A study of the effectiveness of propanolol in menopausal hot flushes. *Br J Obstet Gynaecol* 185:472–75.
10. Crawford, M. P., and Hooper, D. 1973. Menopause, aging and family. *Soc Sci and Med* 7:469–82.
11. Daw, E. 1975. Duration of effect of treatment of menopausal symptoms by oestrogen fraction. *Curr Med Res Opin* 3:22–25.
12. Flint, M. 1975. The menopause: reward or punishment. *Psychosomatics* 16:161–63.
13. Gambrell, R. D. 1977. Postmenopausal bleeding. *Clinics in Obstet & Gynecol* 4:1.
14. Gamst, F. 1969. *The Quemant, a pagan hebraic peasantry of Ethiopia.* New York: Holt, Rinehart and Winston.
15. Guyton, A. C. 1981. *Textbook of medical physiology.* 6th ed. Philadelphia: Saunders.

16. Herold, E.; Mottin, J.; and Sabry, Z. 1979. Effect of vitamin E on human sexual functioning. *Arch Sex Beh* 8:397–403.
17. Hostetler, J., and Huntrington, G. E. 1967. *The Hutterites of North America.* New York: Holt, Rinehart and Winston.
18. Jaszmann, L. J. B. 1973. Epidemiology of climacteric and post climacteric complaints in *Aging and Estrogens* ed. by P. A. Van Keep and C. Lauiritzen. *Front Horm Res* 2:22–34.
19. Kinsey, A.; Pomeroy, W.; and Martin, C. 1953. *Sexual behavior in the human female.* Philadelphia: Saunders.
20. Kronenberg, F.; Carraway, R.; Cote, L. J.; Linkie, D. M.; Crawshaw, L. I.; and Downey, J. A. 1981. Changes in thermoregulation, immunoreactive neurotensin, catecholamines and LH during menopausal hot flashes. In *Proceedings of the sixty-second annual meeting of the American Endocrine Society,* 141, abst. no. 236.
21. Kupperman, H. S.; Wetchler, B. B.; and Blatt, M. H. G. 1959. Contemporary therapy of the menopausal syndrome. *JAMA* 171:1627–37.
22. McKinley, S. M., and Jeffrey, M. 1974. The menopausal syndrome. *Br J Prev Soc Med* 28:108–15.
23. Marks, R., and Shahrad, P. 1977. Skin changes at the time of the climacteric. *Clinics in Obstet & Gynecol* 4:207–26.
24. Meldrum, D.; Tataryn, I.; Frumar, A.; Erlet, J.; Lu, K., and Judd, H. 1980. Gonadotropins, estrogens, and adrenal steroids during the menopausal hot flash. *J Clin Endocrinol Metab* 50:685–89.
25. Metcalf, M. G. 1979. Incidence of ovulatory cycles in women approaching the menopause. *J Biosoc Sci* 11:39–48.
26. Molnar, G. W. 1975. Body temperatures during menopausal hot flashes. *J Appl Physiol* 38:499–503.
27. Molnar, G. W. 1980. Menopausal hot flashes: their cycles and relation to air temperature. *Obstet Gynecol* 57:52S–55S.
28. Punonen, R. 1972. Effect of castration and peroral estrogen therapy on the skin. *Acta Obstet et Gynecol Scand* suppl 21:1–44.
29. Punonen, R., and Rauamo, L. 1977. The effect of long-term oral oestriol succinate therapy on the skin of castrated women. *Ann Chir Gynaecol* 66:214–15.
29a. Semmens, J. P., and Wagner, G. 1982. Estrogen deprivation and vaginal function in postmenopausal women. *JAMA* 248:445–448.
30. Reyes, F.; Winter, J.; and Faiman, C. 1977. Pituitary ovarian relationships preceding the menopause. *Am J Obstet Gynecol* 129:557–64.
31. Ryan, T. J. 1966. The microcirculation of the skin in old age. *Geront Clin* 8:327.
32. Ryan, T. J., and Kurban, A. K. 1970. New vessel growth in the adult skin *Br J Derm* 82, suppl 5:92.
33. Stadel, V., and Weiss, N. 1975. Characteristics of menopausal women: a survey of King and Pierce Counties in Washington, 1973–1974. *Am J Epidemiol* 102:209–216.
34. Studd, J.; Chakravarti, S.; and Oram, D. 1977. The climacteric. *Clinics in Obstet & Gynecol* 4:3–29.

35. Sturdee, D. W.; Wilson, K. A.; Pipili, E.; and Crocker, A. D. 1978. Physiological aspects of menopausal hot flush. *Br Med J* 2:79–80.
36. Tataryn, I. V.; Meldrum, D. R.; Lu, K. H.; Frumar, A. M.; and Judd, H. L. 1979. LH, FSH and skin temperature during the menopause hot flash. *J Clin Endocrinol Metab* 49:152–54.
37. Thompson, B.; Hart, S. A.; and Durno, D. 1973. Menopausal age and symptomatology in a general practice. *J Biosoc Sci* 5:71–82.
38. Thomson, J.; Maddock, J.; Aylward, M.; and Oswald, I. 1977. Relationship between nocturnal plasma oestrogen concentration and free plasma tryptophan in perimenopausal women. *J Endoc* 72:395–96.
39. Thomson, J., and Oswald, I. 1977. Effect of oestrogen on the sleep, mood and anxiety of menopausal women. *Br Med J* 2:317–19.
40. Treloar, A. E. 1974. Menarche, menopause and intervening fecundability. *Human Biology* 16:89–107.
41. ———. 1981. Menstrual cyclicity and the premenopause. *Maturitas* 3:249–64.
42. Treloar, A. E.; Boynton, R. E.; Behn, D. G.; and Brown, B. W. 1967. Variation of the human menstrual cycle through reproductive life. *I J Fertil* 12:77–126.
43. Treloar, A. E.; Boynton, R. E.; and Cowan, D. W. 1974. Secular trend in age at menarche, USA 1893–1974. In *Excerpta Medica international congress series no. 394, biological and clinical aspects of reproduction*. Amsterdam: Excerpta Medica.
44. Vollman, R. F. 1977. *The menstrual cycle*. Major Problems in Obstetrics and Gynecology. Philadelphia: Saunders.

Chapter 3   Body Changes at the Menopause

1. Brown, A. G. 1977. Postmenopausal urinary problems. *Clinics in Obstet & Gynecol* 4:181–206.
2. Costoff, A., and Mahesh, V. B. 1975. Primordial follicles with normal oocytes in the ovaries of postmenopausal women. *J Am Geriatr Soc* 23:193–96.
3. Cutler, W. B., and García, C. R. 1983. Hysterectomy and sexual deficits: a reappraisal and review. In press.
4. Dennefors, B.; Janson, P.; Knutson, F.; and Hamberger, L. 1980. Steroid production and responsiveness to gonadotropin in isolated stromal tissue of human postmenopausal ovaries. *Am J Obstet Gynecol* 136:997–1002.
5. Fedor-Freybergh, P. 1977. The influence of estrogens on the well being and mental performance in climacteric and postmenopausal women. *Acta Obstet et Gynecol Scand* 64: suppl 1–66.
6. Gaddum-Rosse, P.; Rumer, R. E.; Blandau, R. J.; and Theirsch, J. B. 1975. Studies on the mucosa of post menopausal oviducts: surface appearance, ciliary activity and the effect of estrogen treatment. *Fertil Steril* 26:951–69.
7. Kegel, A. M. 1951. Physiologic therapy for urinary stress incontinence. *JAMA* 146: 915–17.

8. Longcope, C.; Hunter, R.; and Franz, C. 1980. Steroid secretion by the post-menopausal ovary. *Am J Obstet Gynecol* 138:564–68.
9. Longcope, C.; Jaffee, W.; and Griffing, G. 1981. Production rates of androgens and oestrogens in postmenopausal women, *Maturitas* 3:215–23.
10. McNatty, K. P.; Makris, A.; DeGrazia, C.; Osathanondh, R.; and Ryan, K. J. 1979. The production of progesterone, androgens and estrogens by granulosa cells, thecal tissue and stromal tissue by human ovaries in vitro. *J Clin Endocrinol Metab* 49: 687–99.
11. Marks, R., and Shahrad, P. 1977. Skin changes at the time of the climacteric. *Clinics in Obstet & Gynecol* 4:207–26.
12. Mikhail, G. 1970. Hormone secretion by the human ovaries. *Gynec Invest* 1:5–20.
13. Monroe, S. E., and Menon, K. M. J. 1977. Changes in reproductive hormone secretion during the climacteric and postmenopausal periods. *Clinics in Obstet & Gynecol* 20:113–22.
14. Novak, E. R. 1970. Ovulation after fifty. *Obstet Gynecol* 36:903–10.
15. Novak, E. R.; Goldberg, B.; and Jones, G. S. 1965. Enzyme histochemistry of the menopausal ovary associated with normal and abnormal endometrium. *Am J Obstet Gynecol* 93:669–73.
16. Novak E. R., and Richardson, E. H. 1941. Proliferative changes in the senile endometrium. *Am J Obstet Gynecol* 42:564.
17. Perry, J. D., and Whipple, B. 1981. Pelvic muscle strength of female ejaculators: evidence in support of a new theory of orgasm. *J Sex Res* 17:22–39.
18. Robertson, D. M., and Landgren, B. M. 1975. Oestradiol receptor levels in the human fallopian tube during the menstrual cycle and after menopause. *J Steroid Biochem* 6:511–13.
19. Rodin, M., and Moghissi, K. S. 1973. Intrinsic innervation of the human cervix: a preliminary study. In *The biology of the human cervix*, ed. R. J. Blandau and K. Moghissi. Chicago: University of Chicago Press.
20. Smith, P. 1972. Age changes in the female urethra. *Br J Urol* 44:667–76.
21. Zussman, L.; Zussman, S.; Sunley, R.; and Bjornson, E. 1981. Sexual response after hysterectomy-oophorectomy: recent studies and reconsideration of psychogenesis. *Am J Obstet Gynecol* 140:725–29.

Chapter 4 The Bones and How They Grow

1. Adams, J. S. 1982. Vitamin D synthesis and metabolism after ultraviolet irradiation of normal and vitamin deficient subjects. *NEJM* 306:722–25.
2. Albanese, A. A. 1978. Calcium nutrition in the elderly. *Postgrad Med* 63:167–72.
3. ———. 1977. Osteoporosis. *J Am Pharm Assoc* 17:252–53.
4. Albanese, A. A.; Edelson, A. H.; Lorenze, E. J.; and Wein, E. H. 1980. Osteoporosis: a new screen for asymptomatic bone loss. *Diagnosis* 2:71.
5. Albanese, A. A.; Edelson, A. A.; Lorenze, E. J.; and Wein, E. H. 1969. Quantitative

radiographic survey technique for the detection of bone loss. *J Am Geriatr Soc* 17:142–54.

6. Albanese, A. A.; Lorenze, E. J.; Edelson, A. H.; Wein, E. H.; and Carroll, L. 1981. Effects of calcium supplements and estrogen replacement therapy on bone loss of postmenopausal women. *Nutrition Reports International* 24:403–14.

7. Albanese, A. A.; Edelson, A. H.; Lorenze, E. J., Jr.; and Woodhull, E. 1975. Problems of bone health in the elderly: a ten year study. *NY State J Med* 75:326–36.

8. Albright, F.; Smith, P. H.; and Richardson, A. M. 1941. Postmenopausal osteoporosis, its clinical features. *JAMA* 116:2465–74.

9. Alfram, P. A. 1964. An epidemiologic study of cervical and trochanteric fractures of the femur in an urban population. *Acta Orthopaedica Scandinavica* 65, suppl. 1: 9–102.

10. Alhava, E. M., and Puittinen, J. 1973. Fractures of the upper end of the femur as an index of senile osteoporosis in Finland. *Ann Clin Res* 5:398 ff.

10a. Beals, R. K. 1972. Survival following hip fracture: long term followup of 607 patients. *J Chron Dis* 25:235–44.

11. Boyle, I. T. 1981. Treatment for postmenopausal osteoporosis. *Lancet* 1376.

12. Bullamore, J. R.; Gallagher, J. C.; and Wilkinson, R. 1970. Effect of age on calcium absorption. *Lancet* 2:535–37.

13. Chalmers, J., and Ho, K. C. 1970. Geographical variations in senile osteoporosis: the association with physical activity. *J Bone and Joint Surgery* 52b:667–75.

14. Chestnut, C. H. 1981. Treatment of postmenopausal osteoporosis: some current concepts. *Scott Med J* 26:72 ff.

15. Chestnut, C. H.; Baylink, D. J.; and Nelp, W. B. 1979. Calcitonin therapy in postmenopausal osteoporosis: preliminary results. *Clin Res* 27:85A abstract.

16. Christianssen, C., and Christensen, M. S. 1981. Bone mass in postmenopausal women after withdrawal of oestrogen/gestagen replacement therapy. *Lancet* 459–61.

17. Crilly, R.; Horsman, A.; Marshall, D. H.; and Nordin, B. E. C. 1979. Prevalence, pathogenesis and treatment of post-menopausal osteoporosis. *Aust N Z J Med* 9: 24–30.

18. Gallagher, J., and Nordin, B. E. C. 1975. Effects of oestrogen and progestogen therapy on calcium metabolism in post-menopausal women. *Front Horm Res* 3:150.

19. Gallagher, J. C.; Riggs, B. L.; and DeLuca, H. F. 1978. Effect of age on calcium absorption and serum 1,25 OH2D. *Clin Res* 26:680A.

20. Garn, S. M. 1970. *The earlier gain and the later loss of cortical bone in nutritional perspective.* Springfield, Ill.: Charles C. Thomas.

21. Geola, F.; Frumar, A.; Tataryn, I.; Lu, K.; Hershman, J.; Eggena, P.; Sambhi, M.; and Judd, H. 1980. Biological effects of various doses of conjugated equine estrogens in postmenopausal women. *J Clin Endocrinol Metab* 51:620–25.

22. Gordan, G. S. 1981. Early detection of osteoporosis and prevention of hip fractures in elderly women. *Med Times* special section (April), pp. 1s–17s.

23. Heaney, R. P. 1962. Radiocalcium metabolism in disuse osteoporosis in man. *Amer J Med* 33:188–200.

24. Heaney, R. P.; Recker, R. R.; and Saville, P. D. 1977. Calcium balance and calcium requirements in middle aged women. *Am J Clin Nutr* 30:1603.

25. Hempel, Von E.; Kriester, A.; Freesmeyer, E.; and Walter, W. 1979. Perspecktive studie zur osteoporose nach bilater ovarektomie mit und ohne postoperative ostregenprophylaxe. *Zentralblatt für Gynakologie* 101:309–19.

26. Ireland, P., and Fordtran, J. S. 1973. Effect of dietary calcium on age on jejunal calcium absorption in humans studied by intestinal perfusion. *J Clin Invest* 52: 2672–81.

27. Lafferty, F. W.; Spencer, G. E.; and Pearson, O. H. 1964. Effects of androgens, estrogens and high calcium intakes on bone formation and resorption in osteoporosis. *Am J Med* 36:514–28.

28. Lee, C. J.; Lawler, G. S.; and Johnson, G. H. 1981. Effects of supplementation of the diets with calcium and calcium rich foods on bone density of elderly females with osteoporosis. *Am J Clin Nutr* 34:819–23.

29. Lindsay, R.; Aitken, J. M.; and Anderson, J. B. 1976. Long term prevention of postmenopausal osteoporosis by estrogen. *Lancet* 1:1038–40.

30. Lindsay, R.; Aitken, J. M.; Hart, D. M.; and Purdie, D. 1978. The effect of ovarian sex steroids on bone mineral status in the oophorectomized rat and in the human. *Postgrad Med J* 54:50–58.

31. Marshall, D. H.; Crilly, R. G.; and Nordin, B. E. 1977. Plasma androstenedione and oestrone levels in normal and osteoporotic postmenopausal women. *Br Med J* 2: 1177–79.

32. Meema, H. E.; Bunker, M. I.; and Meema, S. 1965. Loss of compact bone due to menopause. *Obstet Gynecol* 26:333–38.

33. Meema, S., and Meema, H. E. 1976. Menopausal bone loss and estrogen replacement. *Israel J Med Sci* 12:601–6.

34. Meunier, P.; Courpron, P.; Edourd, C.; Bernard, J.; Bringuier, J.; and Vignon, E. 1973. Physiological senile involution and pathological rarefaction of bone. *Clin Endocrinol Metab* 2:239–56.

35. Nachtigall, L. E.; Nachtigall, R. H.; Nachtigall, R. D.; and Beckman, E. M. 1979. Estrogen replacement therapy 1: a 10 year prospective study in the relationship to osteoporosis. *Obstet Gynecol* 53:277–81.

36. Nordin, B. E. C.; Gallagher, J. C.; Aaron, J. E.; and Horsman, H. 1975. Postmenopausal osteopenia and osteoporosis. *Estrogens in the postmenopause*. Vol. 3 of *Frontiers in hormone research*. Basel: Karger.

37. Nordin, B. E. C.; Horsman, A.; Marshall, D. H.; Simpson, M.; and Waterhouse, G. M. 1979. Calcium requirement and calcium therapy. *Clin Orthop and Rel Res* 140:216–39.

38. Rasmussen, H.; Bordier, P.; Marie, P.; Auguier, L.; Eisinger, J. B.; Kuntz, D.; Caulin, F.; Argemi, B.; Gueris, J.; and Julien, A. 1980. Effect of combined therapy with phosphate and calcitonin on bone volume in osteoporosis. *Metab Bone Dis & Rel Res* 2:107–11.

39. Reynolds, J. J.; Holick, M. F.; and DeLuca, H. H. F. 1973. The role of vitamin D metabolites in bone resorption. *Calcif Tissue Res* 12:295–301.

40. Riggs, B. L.; Hodgson, S. F.; Hoffman, D. L.; Kelly, P. J.; Johnson, K. A.; and Taves, D. 1980. Treatment of primary osteoporosis with fluoride and calcium. *JAMA* 243: 446.
41. Riggs, B. L.; Seeman, E.; Hodgson, S. F.; Taves, D. R.; and O'Fallon, W. M. 1982. Effect of the fluoride/calcium regimen on vertebral fracture occurrence in post-menopausal osteoporosis. *NEJM* 306:446–50.
42. Smith, D. M.; Khairi, M. R. A.; Norton, J.; and Johnston, C. C., Jr. 1976. Age and activity effects on rate of bone mineral loss. *J Clin Invest* 568:716–21.
43. Urist, M. R. 1973. Orthopedic management of postmenopausal osteoporosis. *Clin Endocrinol Metab* 2:159–76.
44. Watson, R. C. 1973. Bone growth and physical activity. In *International conference on bone mineral measurements*, 380–85.

ADDITIONAL RECOMMENDED READINGS

Aitken, J. M.; Hart, D. M.; and Lindsay, R. 1973. Oestrogen replacement therapy for prevention of osteoporosis after oophorectomy. *Br Med J* 3:515–18.

Brown, D. J.; Spanos, E.; and MacIntyre, I. 1980. Role of pituitary hormones in regulating renal vitamin D metabolism in man. *Br Med J* 1:277–78.

Cann, C. E.; Genant, H. K.; Ettinger, B.; and Gordan, G. S. 1980. Spinal mineral loss of quantitative computed tomography in oophorectomized women. *JAMA* 244: 2056–59.

Crilly, R. G.; Marshall, D. H.; and Nordin, B. E. 1979. Effect of age on plasma andros-tenedione concentration in oophorectomized women. *Clin Endocrinol (Oxf)* 10: 199–201.

Dalen, N., and Olsson, K. E. 1974. Bone mineral content and physical activity. *Acta Orthopaedica Scandinavia* 45:170–74.

Daniell, H. W. 1976. Osteoporosis of the slender smoker. *Arch Intern Med* 136:298 ff.

Deftos, L. J.; Roos, B. A.; Bronzert, D.; and Parthemore, J. G. 1975. Immunochemical heterogeneity of calcitonin in plasma. *Clinical Endocrinol Metab* 40:409–12.

Deftos, L. J., and Weisman, M. H. 1980. Influence of age and sex on plasma calcitonin in human beings. *NEJM* 40:409–12.

Gallagher, J. C.; Aaron, J.; Horsman, A.; Marshall, D. H.; Wilkinson, R.; and Nordin, B. E. C. 1973. The crush fracture syndrome in postmenopausal women. *Clin Endo-crinol Metab* 2:293.

Gallagher, J. C.; Horsman, A.; and Nordin, B. E. C. 1974. Osteoporosis in the menopause. In *The menopausal syndrome*, ed. R. B. Greenblatt, V. B. Mahesh, and P. G. McDonough. New York: Medcom Press.

Gallagher, J. C.; Melton, L. J.; Riggs, B. L.; and Bergstrath, E. 1980. Epidemiology of fractures of the proximal femur in Rochester, Minnesota, USA. *Clin Orthop* 150: 163–71.

Girgis, S. I.; Hillyard, C. J.; MacIntyre, I.; and Szelke, M., eds. 1977. *An immunological comparison of normal circulating calcitonin with calcitonin from medullary carcinoma.* Amsterdam: Elsevier North-Holland Biomedical Press.

Goldsmith, N. F. 1971. Bone-mineral estimation in normal and osteoporotic women: a comparability trial of four methods and seven bone sites. *J Bone Joint Surg (AM)* 53A:83–100.

Heaney, R. P. 1974. Pathophysiology of osteoporosis: implication for treatment. *Tex Med* 70:37–45.

Heath, H., and Sizemore, G. 1977. Plasma calcitonin in normal man. *J Clin Invest* 60:1135–40.

Hillyard, C. J.; Stevenson, J. C.; and MacIntyre, I. 1978. Relative deficiency of plasma-calcitonin in normal women. *Lancet* 961–62.

Horsman, A.; Gallagher, J. C.; Simpson, M.; and Nordin, B. E. C. 1977. Prospective trial of oestrogen and calcium in postmenopausal women. *Br Med J* 2:789–92.

Horsman, A.; Nordin, B. E. C.; Gallagher, J. C.; Kirby, P. A.; Milner, R. M.; and Simpson, M. 1977. Observations of sequential changes in bone mass in post-menopausal women: a controlled trial of oestrogen and calcium therapy. *Calif Tiss Res* suppl. 22:217–24.

Hutchinson, T. A.; Polansy, S. M.; and Feinstein, A. R. 1979. Postmenopausal estrogens protect against fractures of hip and distal radius, a case-control study. *Lancet* 2: 705–9.

Lindsay, R.; Hart, D. M.; MacLean, A.; Clark, A. C.; Kraszewski, A.; and Garwood, J. 1978. Bone response to termination of oestrogen treatment. *Lancet* 1:1325–27.

Longcope, C.; Jafee, W.; and Griffin, G. 1981. Production rates of androgens and oestrogens in postmenopausal women. *Maturitas* 3:215–23.

MacIntyre, I.; Evans, I. M. A.; Hobitz, H. H. G.; Joplin, G. F.; and Stevenson, J. C. 1980. Chemistry, physiology, and therapeutic applications of calcitonin. *Arthritis and Rheumatism* 23:1139–47.

MacIntyre, I., and Parsons, J. A. 1967. The effect of thyrocalcitonin on blood bone calcium equilibrium in the perfused tibia of the cat. *J Physiol (London)* 191:393–405.

Marshall, D. H.; Crilly, R.; and Nordin, B. E. 1978. The relation between plasma androstenedione and oestrone levels in untreated and corticosteroid treated postmenopausal women. *Clin Endocrinol (Oxf)* 9:407–12.

Marshall, D. H., and Nordin, B. E. 1977. The effect of 1 alpha-hydroxyvitamin D3 with and without oestrogens on calcium balance in postmenopausal women. *Clin Endocrinol (Oxf)* 7, suppl.: 159s–68s.

Martin, P. 1982. Unpublished data.

Nilson, B. E., and Westlin, N. E. 1971. Bone density in athletes. *Clin Orthop and Rel Res* 77:179–82.

Pak, C. Y. C.; Stewart, A.; Kaplan, R.; Bone, H.; Notz, C.; and Browne, R. 1975. Photon absorptiometric analysis of bone density in primary hyperparathyroidism. *Lancet* 2:7–8.

Rasmussen, H., and Bordier, P. 1974. *The physiological basis of metabolic bone disease.* Baltimore: Williams & Wilkins.

Recker, R. R.; Saville, P. C.; and Heaney, R. P. 1977. Effect of estrogens and calcium carbonate on bone loss in postmenopausal women. *Ann Int Med* 87:649–55.

Riggs, B. L.; Jowsey, J.; Goldsmith, R. S.; Kelly, P. J.; Hoffman, D. L.; and Arnaud, C. D. 1972. Short and long-term effects of estrogen and synthetic anabolic hormone in postmenopausal osteoporosis. *J Clin Invest* 51:1659–63.

Riggs, B. L.; Jowsey, J.; Kelly, P. J.; Jones, J. D.; and Maher, F. T. 1969. Effect of sex hormones on bone in primary osteoporosis. *J Clin Invest* 48:1065.

Samaan, N., and Anderson, G. D. 1975. Immunoreactive calcitonin in the mother, neonate, child and adult. *Am J Obstet Gynecol* 121:622–25.

Smith, E. L., and Reddan, W. 1976. Physical activity—a modality for bone accretion in the aged: conference on bone mineral measurement. *Am J Roentgenology* 126: 1297.

Smith, E. L.; Reddan, W.; and Smith, P. E. 1981. Physical activity and calcium modalities of bone mineral increase in aged women. *Med Sci Sports and Exercise* 13:60–64.

Stevenson, J. C. 1980. The structure and function of calcitonin. *Investigations and Cell Path* 3:187–93.

Stevenson, J. C.; Hillyard, C. J.; Abeyasekara, G.; Phang, K. G.; MacIntyre, I.; Campbell, S.; Young, O.; Townsend, P. T.; and Whitehead, M. I. 1981. Calcitonin and the calcium-regulating hormones in postmenopausal women: effect of estrogens. *Lancet* 693–95.

Stevenson, J. C., and Whitehead, M. I. 1982. Calcitonin secretion and postmenopausal osteoporosis. *Lancet* 804.

Taggart, H.; Ivey, J. L.; Sison, K.; Chestnut, C. H., III; Baylink, D. J.; Huber, M. B.; and Roos, B. A. 1982. Deficient calcitonin response to calcium stimulation in post-menopausal osteoporosis. *Lancet* 475.

Wallach, S., and Henneman, P. H. 1959. Prolonged estrogen therapy in postmenopausal women. *JAMA* 171:1637.

Whyte, M. P.; Bergfeld, M. A.; Murphy, W. A.; Avioli, L. V.; and Teitelbaum, S. L. 1982. Postmenopausal osteoporosis: a heterogeneous disorder as assessed by histomorphometric analysis of iliac crest bone from untreated patients. *Am J Med* 72:193–202.

Wiske, P. S.; Epstein, N. H.; Bell, N. H.; Queener, S. F.; Edmondson, J.; and Johnston, C. C. 1979. Increases in immunoreactive parathyroid hormone with age. *NEJM* 300:1419–21.

Chapter 5   Hormone Replacement Therapy I

1. Aitken, J. M.; Hart, D. M.; and Lindsay, R. 1973. Oestrogen replacement therapy for prevention of osteoporosis after oophorectomy. *Br Med J* 3:515–18.
2. Bancroft, J.; Davidson, D. W.; Warner, P.; and Tyrer, G. 1979. Androgens and sexual behavior in women using oral contraceptives. *Clin Endocrinol*
3. Bolton, C. H.; Ellwood, M.; Hartog, M.; Martin, R.; Rowe, A. S.; and Wensley, R. T. 1975. Comparison of the effects of ethinyl oestradiol and conjugated equine oestrogens in oophorectomized women. *Clin Endocrinol (Oxf)* 4:131–38.

4. Brown, A. G. 1977. Postmenopausal urinary problems. *Clinics in Obstet & Gynecol* 4:181–206.

5. Burnier, A. M.; Martin, P. L.; Yen, S. S. C.; and Brooks, P. 1981. Sublingual absorption of micronized 17β estradiol. *Am J Obstet Gynecol* 140:146–50.

6. Burns, D. D., and Mendels, J. 1979. Serotonin and affective disorders. In *Current developments in psychopharmacology*, ed. W. B. Easman and L. Valzelli, pp. 293–359. Vol 5. New York: SP Medical and Scientific Books.

6a. Bush, T. L.; Cowan, L. D.; Barrett-Connor, E.; Criqui, M. H.; Karon, J. M.; Wallace, R. B.; Tyroler, H. A.; and Rifkind, B. M. 1983. Estrogen use and all-cause mortality. *JAMA* 249:903–6.

7. Byrd, B. F.; Burch, J. C.; and Vaughn, W. K. 1977. The impact of long term estrogen support after hysterectomy: a report of 1016 cases. *Ann Surg* 185:574–80.

8. Campbell, S., and Whitehead, M. 1977. Oestrogen therapy and the menopausal syndrome. *Clinics in Obstet & Gynecol* 4:31–47.

9. Cutler, W. C.; Davidson, J. M.; and McCoy, N. 1983. Sexual behavior frequency and absence of hot flashes are associated. In preparation.

10. Deghengh, R. 1979. Chemistry and biochemistry of natural estrogens. In *The menopause and post menopause: proceedings of an international symposium*, ed. N. Pasetto, R. Paoletti, and J. L. Ambrus, pp. 3–16. England: MTP Press.

11. Dennerstein, L.; Burrows, G. D.; and Hyman, G. 1979. Hormone therapy and affect. *Maturitas* 1:247–59.

12. Deutch, S.; Ossowski, R.; and Benjamin, I. 1981. Comparison between degree of systemic absorption of vaginally and orally administered estrogens at different dose levels in post menopausal women. *Am J Obstet Gynecol* 139:967–68.

13. Englund, D. E., and Johansson, E. D. B. 1980. Endometrial effect of oral estriol treatment in postmenopausal women. *Acta Obstet et Gynecol Scand* 59:449–51.

14. Fedor-Freybergh, P. 1977. The influence of estrogens on the well-being and mental performance in the climacterica and postmenopausal women. *Acta Obstet et Gynecol Scand* 64, suppl. 1:1–66.

15. Feigen, G. A.; Fraser, R. C.; and Peterson, N. W. 1978. Sex hormones and the immune response II: perturbation of antibody production by estradiol 17β. *Int Arch Allergy Appl Immunol* 57:488–97.

16. Gambrell, R. D. 1982. The menopause: benefits and risks of estrogen-progestogen replacement therapy. *Fertil Steril* 4:457–74.

16a. García, C. R., and Drill, V. A. 1977. Contraceptive steroids and liver lesions. *J Toxicol Environ Health* 3:197–206.

17. Geola, F.; Frumar, A.; Tataryn, I.; Lu, K.; Hershman, J.; Eggena, P.; Sambhi, M.; and Judd, H. 1980. Biological effects of various doses of conjugated equine estrogens in postmenopausal women. *J Clin Endocrinol Metab* 51:620–25.

18. Gordan, W. E.; Herman, H. W.; and Hunter, D. C. 1979. Treatment of atrophic vaginitis in postmenopausal women with micronized estradiol cream—a follow up study. *J Kentucky Med Assn* 77:337–19.

19. Haspels, A. A.; Bennink, J. H.; VanKeep, P. A.; and Schreurs, W. H. 1975. Estrogens and vitamin B6. *Front Horm Res* 3:199–207.

20. Haspels, A. A.; Coelingh Bennink, H. J. T.; and Schreurs, W. H. P. 1978. Disturbance of tryptophan metabolism and its correction during oestrogen treatment in postmenopausal women. *Maturitas* 1:15–20.

21. Hasselquist, M.; Goldberg, N.; Schroeter, A.; and Spelsbert, T. 1980. Isolation and characterization of the estrogen receptor in human skin. *J Clin Endocrinol Metab* 50:76–82.

22. Kegel, A. M. 1951. Physiologic therapy for urinary stress incontinence. *JAMA* 146: 915–17.

23. Kupperman, H. S.; Wetchler, B. B.; and Blatt, M. H. G. 1959. Contemporary therapy for the menopausal syndrome. *JAMA* 171:1627–37.

24. Larsson-Cohn, U.; Johansson, E.; Kagedal, B.; and Wallentin, L. 1977. Serum FSH, LH and oestrone levels in postmenopausal patients on oestrogen therapy. *Br J Obstet Gynaecol* 86:367–72.

25. Lauritzen, C. 1973. The management of the premenopausal and the postmenopausal patient. *Front Horm Res* 2:2–21.

26. Martin, P.; Yen, S. S. C.; Burnier, A. M.; and Hermann, H. 1979. Systemic absorption and sustained effects of vaginal estrogen creams. *JAMA* 242:2699–2700.

27. Nielson, F. H.; Honore, E.; Kristoffersen, K.; Secher, N. J.; and Pederson, G. T. 1977. Changes in serum lipids during treatment with norgestrel, oestradiol-valerate and cycloprogynon. *Acta Obstet et Gynecol Scand* 56:367–70.

28. Pallas, K. G.; Holzwarth, G. J.; Stern, M. P.; and Lucas, C. P. 1977. The effects of conjugated estrogen on the renin-angiotensin system. *J Clin Endocrinol Metab* 44: 1061–68.

29. Punonen, R. 1972. Effect of castration and peroral estrogen therapy on the skin. *Acta Obstet et Gynecol Scand* suppl 21:1–44.

30. Punonen, R.; Lammintausta, R.; Erkkola, R.; Rauramo, L. 1980. Estradiol valerate therapy and the renin-aldosterone system in castrated women. *Maturitas* 2:91–94.

31. Punonen, R., and Rauramo, L. 1977. The effect of long-term oral oestriol succinate therapy on the skin of castrated women. *Ann Chir Gynaecol* 66:214–15.

32. Rigg, L. A.; Hermann, H.; and Yen, S. S. C. 1977. Absorption of estrogens from vaginal creams. *NEJM* 242:2699–2700.

33. Rose, D. P. 1966. Excretion of xanthurenic acid in the urine of women taking progestogen-oestrogen preparations. *Nature* 210:196–97.

34. Schiff, I., and Ryan, K. 1980. Benefits of estrogen replacement. *Obstet & Gynecol Survey* 35:400–11.

35. Schiff, I.; Tulchinsky, D.; and Ryan, K. J. 1977. Vaginal absorption of estrogen and 17β estradiol. *Fertil Steril* 23:1063–66.

36. Schiff, I.; Wentworth, B.; Koos, B.; Ryan, K. J.; and Tulchinsky, D. 1978. Effect of estriol administration on the hypogonadal woman. *Fertil Steril* 30:278–82.

37. Schneider, M. A.; Brotherton, P. L.; and Hailes, J. 1977. The effect of exogenous oestrogens on depression in menopausal women. *Med J Aust* 2:162–63.

37a. Semmens, J. P., and Wagner, G. 1982. Estrogen deprivation and vaginal function in post menopausal women. *JAMA* 248:445–48.

38. Stark, M.; Adonia, A.; Milwidsky, A.; Gilon, G.; and Palti, Z. 1978. Can estrogens

218 BIBLIOGRAPHY

be useful for treatment of vaginal relaxation in elderly women? *Am J Obstet Gynecol* 131:585–86.

39. Studd, J. W. W.; Collins, W. P.; Chakravarti, S.; Newton, J. R.; Oram, D.; and Parsons, A. 1977. Oestradiol and testosterone implants in the treatment of psychosexual problems in the postmenopausal woman. *Br J Obstet Gynaecol* 84:314–16.

40. Thomson, J.; Maddock, J.; Aylward, M.; and Oswald, I. 1977. Relationship between nocturnal plasma oestrogen concentration and free plasma tryptophan in postmenopausal women. *J Endoc* 72:395–96.

41. Thomson, J., and Oswald, I. 1977. Effect of oestrogen on the sleep, mood and anxiety of menopausal women. *Br Med J* 2:317–19.

42. VanKeep, P. A.; Serr, D. M.; Greenblatt, R. B.; and Kopera, H. 1978. Effects, side effects, and dosage schemes of various sex hormones in the peri and post menopause. Worshop report in *Female and male climacteric: current opinion 1978*. Baltimore: University Park Press.

Chapter 6   Hormone Replacement Therapy II

1. Buchman, M. I.; Kramer, E.; and Felman, G. B. 1978. Aspiration curettage for asymptomatic patients receiving estrogen. *Obstet Gynecol* 51:339–41.

2. Budoff, P. W., and Sommers, J. C. 1979. Estrogen progesterone therapy in postmenopausal women. *J Reprod Med* 22:241–47.

3. Campbell, S.; Minardi, J.; McQueen, J.; and Whitehead, M. 1978. Endometrial factors: the modifying effect of progestogen on the response of the postmenopausal endometrium to exogenous estrogens. *Postgrad Med J* 54:59–64.

4. Denis, R.; Barnett, J. M.; and Forbes, S. E. 1973. Diagnostic suction curettage. *Obstet Gynecol* 42:301–3.

5. *Dorland's illustrated medical dictionary*. 1974. 25th ed. Philadelphia: Saunders.

6. Flickinger, G. L.; Elsner, C.; Illingworth, D. V.; Muechler, E. K.; and Mikhail, G. 1977. Estrogen and progesterone receptors in the female genital tract of humans and monkeys. *Ann NY Academy of Sciences* 286:180–89.

7. Gambrell, R. D. 1982. The menopause: benefits and risks of estrogen-progestogen replacement therapy. *Fertil Steril* 37:457–74.

8. Gambrell, R. D., Jr. 1982. Role of hormones in the etiology and prevention of endometrial and breast cancer. *Acta Obstet et Gynecol Scand* suppl 106:37–46.

9. ———. 1977. Postmenopausal bleeding. *Clinics in Obstet & Gynecol* 4:1.

10. Gambrell, R. D., Jr.; Castaneda, T. A.; and Ricci, C. A. 1978. Management of postmenopausal bleeding to prevent endometrial cancer. *Maturitas* 1:99–106.

11. Gambrell, R. D., Jr.; Massey, F. M.; Castaneda, T. A.; Ugenas, A. J.; Ricci, C. A.; and Wright, J. M. 1980. Use of progestogen challenge test to reduce the risk of endometrial cancer. *Obstet Gynecol* 55:732–38.

12. Gordon, J.; Reagan, J. W.; Finkle, W. D.; and Ziel, H. K. 1977. Estrogen and endometrial carcinoma: independent pathology review supporting original risk estimate. *NEJM* 297:570–71.

13. Gurpide, E.; Gusberg, S. B.; and Tseng, L. 1976. Oestradiol binding and metabolism in human endometrial hyperplasia and adenocarcinoma. *J Steroid Biochem* 7:891–96.
14. Gusberg, S. B. 1976. The individual at high risk for endometrial carcinoma. *Am J Obstet Gynecol* 126:535.
15. ———. 1975. A strategy for the control of endometrial cancer. *Proc Royal Soc of Med* 68:163–68.
16. Guyton, A. C. 1981. *Textbook of medical physiology.* 6th ed. Philadelphia: Saunders.
17. Hammond, C. B. 1980. Progestins with estrogen replacement curb cancer risk. *Ob/ Gyn News,* Sept. 15, pp. 4–5.
18. Hammond, C. B.; Jelovsek, F. R.; Lee, K. L.; Creasman, W. T.; and Parker, R. T. 1979. Effects of long term estrogen replacement therapy II: neoplasia. *Am J Obstet Gynecol* 133:537–47.
19. Hoover, R.; Gray, L. A.; Cole, P.; and MacMahon, B. 1976. Menopausal estrogens and breast cancer. *NEJM* 295:401–5.
20. Hulka, B. 1980. Effect of exogenous estrogen on postmenopausal women: the epidemiologic evidence. *Obstet & Gynecol Survey* 35:389–99.
21. Hutton, J. D.; Morse, A. R.; Anderson, M. C.; and Beard, R. W. 1978. Endometrial assessment with Isaacs Cell Sampler. *Br Med J* 1:947–49.
22. Jones, G. 1966. Sexual difficulties after 50: gynecological comments. *Obstet & Gynecol Survey* 21:628.
23. Jordan, J. A. 1980. Is death from cervical cancer avoidable? *Royal Soc of Health J* 100:231–33.
24. Kay, C. R. 1978. Logistics of study on hormone therapy in the climacteric. *Postgrad Med J* 2:92–94.
25. King, R. J.; Whitehead, M. I.; Campbell, S.; and Minardi, J. 1978. Biochemical studies of endometrium from postmenopausal women receiving hormone replacement therapy. *Postgrad Med J* 54:65–68.
26. Kupperman, H. S.; Wetchler, B. B.; and Blatt, M. H. G. 1959. Contemporary therapy for the menopausal syndrome. *JAMA* 171:1627–37.
27. Larsson-Cohn, U.; Johansson, E.; Kagedal, B.; and Wallentin, L. 1977. Serum FSH, LH and oestrone levels in postmenopausal patients on oestrogen therapy. *Br J Obstet Gynaecol* 85:367–72.
28. Ludwig, N. 1982. The morphologic response of the human endometrium to long-term treatment with progestational agents. *Am J Obstet Gynecol* 142:796–808.
29. McBride, J. M. 1959. Premenopausal cystic glandular hyperplasia and endometrial carcinoma. *J Ob Gyn of the Br Commonwealth* 66:288 ff.
30. McDonald, T. W.; Annegers, J. F.; and O'Fallon, W. M. 1977. Exogenous estrogen and endometrial carcinoma. *Am J. Obstet Gynecol* 127:572–80.
31. MacMahon, B. 1974. Risk factors for endometrial cancer. *Gynecol Oncol* 2:122–29.
32. Menczer, J.; Modan, M.; Ezra, D.; and Serr, D. M. 1980. Prognosis in pre- and post-menopausal patients with endometrial adenocarcinoma. *Maturitas* 2:37–44.
33. Mickal, A., and Torres, J. 1974. Adenocarcinoma of endometrium. In *The menopausal syndrome,* ed. R. B. Greenblatt, V. B. Mahesh, and P. G. McDonough. New York: Medcome Press.

34. Ng, A. B. P., and Reagan, J. W. 1970. Incidence and prognosis of endometrial carcinoma by histologic grade and extent. *Obstet Gynecol* 35:437–42.
35. Ng, A.B. P.; Reagan, J. W.; Storaasli, J. P.; and Wentz, W. B. 1973. Mixed adenosquamos carcinoma of the endometrium, *Am J of Clin Pathol* 59:765–81.
36. Paterson, M. E. L.; Wade-Evans, T.; Sturdee, D. W.; Thom, M. H.; and Studd, J. W. W. 1980. Endometrial disease after treatment with oestrogens and progestogens in the climacteric. *Br. Med J* 96:1–8.
37. Reagan, J. W., and Ng, A. B. P. 1973. *The cells of uterine adenocarcinoma.* 2d ed. Basel: Kargel.
38. Rosenfeld, D. L., and García, C.-R. 1975. Endometrial biopsy in the cycle of conception. *Fertil Steril* 26:1088–93.
39. Ross, R. K.; Paganini-Hill, A.; Gerkins, V. R.; Mack, T. M.; et al. 1980. A case control study of menopausal estrogen therapy and breast cancer. *JAMA* 243:1635.
40. Schiff, I., and Ryan, K. 1980. Benefits of estrogen replacement. *Obstet & Gynecol Survey* 35:400–11.
41. Stahl, N. L. 1974. Hormones and cancer. In *The menopausal syndrome*, ed. R. B. Greenblatt, V. B. Mahesh, and P. G. McDonough. New York: Medcome Press.
42. Sturdee, D. W.; Wade-Evans, T.; Paterson, M. E.; Thom, M.; and Studd, J. W. 1978. Relations between bleeding pattern, endometrial histology, and oestrogen treatment in menopausal women. *Br. Med J* 1:1575–77.
43. Tseng, L., and Gurpide, E. 1973. Effect of estrone and progesterone on the nuclear uptake of estradiol by slices of endometrium. *Endocrinol* 93:245–48.
44. Valle, R. F. 1981. Hysteroscopic evaluation of patients with abnormal uterine bleeding. *Surg Gynecol Obstet* 153:521–26.
45. Vanderick, C.; Beernaert, J.; and DeMuylder, E. 1975. Hormonal contraception, sequential formulations and the endometrium. *Contraception* 12:655–664.
46. VanKeep, P. A.; Serr, D. M.; Greenblatt, R. B.; and Kopera, H. 1978. Effects, side effects, and dosage schemes of various sex hormones in the peri and post menopause. Worshop report in *Female and male climacteric: current opinion 1978.* Baltimore: University Park Press.
47. Waldron, I. 1982. An analysis of causes of sex differences in mortality and morbidity. In *The fundamental connection between nature and nurture*, ed. W. R. Gove and G. R. Carpenter. Lexington, Mass.: Lexington Books.
48. Weiss, N. J. 1975. Risks and benefits of estrogen use. *NEJM* 293:1200–2.
49. Wentz, W. B. 1974. Progestin therapy in endometrial hyperplasia. *Gynecol Oncol* 2:362–67.
50. Whitehead, M. I.; McQueen, J.; Minardi, J.; and Campbell, S. 1978. Clinical considerations in the management of the menopause: the endometrium. *Postgrad Med J* 54:69–73.
51. Whitehead, M. I.; Townsend, P. T.; Pryse-Davies, J.; Ryder, T. A.; and King, R. J. B. 1981. Effects of estrogens and progestins on the biochemistry and morphology of the postmenopausal endometrium. *NEJM* 305:1599–1605.
52. Whitehead, M. I.; Townsend, P. T.; Pryse-Davies, J.; Ryder, T.; Lane, G.; Soddle, N.; and King, R. J. B. 1982. Actions of progestins on the morphology and biochemis-

try of the endometrium of postmenopausal women receiving low-dose estrogen therapy. *Am J Obstet Gynecol* 142:791–95.

53. Whitehead, M. I.; Townsend P. T.; Pryse-Davies, J.; Ryder, T.; Lane, G.; Soddle, N.; King, R. J. B. 1982. Actions of progestins on the morphology and biochemistry of the endometrium of postmenopausal women receiving low-dose estrogen therapy. *Am J Obstet Gynecol* 142:791–95.

54. Wynder, E. L.; Eschjer, G. C.; and Matnel, N. 1966. An epidemiological investigation of cancer of the endometrium. *Cancer* 19:489–520.

55. Ziel, H. K., and Finkle, W. D. 1975. Increased risk of endometrial carcinoma among users of conjugated estrogens. *NEJM* 293:1167–70.

ADDITIONAL RECOMMENDED READINGS

Abramson, D., and Driscoll, S. G. 1966. Endometrial aspiration biopsy. *Obstet Gynecol* 27:381–91.

Botella Llusia, J.; Oriol-Bosch, A.; Sanchez-Garrido, F.; and Tresquerres, J. A. F. 1980. Testosterone and 17 β oestradiol secretion of the human ovary, II: normal postmenopausal women, postmenopausal women with endometrial hyperplasia and postmenopausal women with adenocarcinoma of the endometrium. *Maturitas* 2:7–12.

Callantine, M. R.; Martin, P. L.; Bolding, O. T.; Warner, P. O.; and Greaney, M. O., Jr. 1975. Micronized 17 beta estradiol for oral estrogen therapy in menopausal women. *Obstet Gynecol* 46:37–41.

Campbell, S., and Whitehead, M. 1977. Oestrogen therapy and the menopausal syndrome. *Clinics in Obstet & Gynecol* 4:31–47.

Centaro, A.; Ceci, G.; de Laurentis, G.; and de Salvia, D. 1974. Epidemiologic studies of postmenopausal endometrial adenocarcinoma. In *The menopausal syndrome*, ed. R. B. Greenblatt, V. B. Mahesh, and P. G. McDonough, pp. 133–38. New York: Medcome Press.

Horwitz, R. I.; Feinstein, A. R.; Horwitz, S. M.; and Robboy, S. J. 1981. Necropsy diagnosis of endometrial cancer and detection bias in case/control studies. *Lancet* 66–67.

Horwitz, R. I., and Feinstein, A. R. 1978. Alternative analytic methods for case control studies of estrogens and endometrial cancer. *NEJM* 299:1089–94.

Tseng, L.; Stolee, A.; and Gurpide, E. 1972. Quantitative studies on the uptake and metabolism of estrogens and progesterone by human endometrium. *Endocrinol* 90:390–404.

Van Campehout, J.; Choquette, P.; and Vauclair, P. 1980. Endometrial pattern in patients with primary hypoestrogenic amenorrhea receiving estrogen replacement therapy. *Obstet Gynecol* 56:349–55.

Chapter 7   Sexuality in the Menopausal Years

1. Abramov, L. 1976. Sexual life and frigidity among women developing acute myocardial infarction. *Psychosomatic Medicine* 38:418–25.
2. Adams, D. B.; Gold, A. R.; and Burt, A. D. 1978. Rise in female-initiated sexual activity at ovulation and its suppression by oral contraceptives. *NEJM* 299:1145–50.
3. Bancroft, J.; Davidson, D. W.; Warner, P.; and Tyrer, G. 1979. Androgens and sexual behavior of women using oral contraceptives. *Clin Endocrinol* 12:327–40.
4. Bancroft, J., and Skakkeback, N. S. 1978. Androgens and human sexual behavior. 209–20. In *CIBA Foundation symposium, 62. Sex, hormones and behavior.* Amsterdam: Excerpta Medica.
5. Christenson, C. V., and Johnson, A. B. 1973. Sexual patterns in a group of older never-married women. *J Geriatr Psychiatry* 7:80–98.
6. Cutler, W. B.; Davidson, J. M.; and McCoy, N. 1983. Sexual behavior frequency and hot flashes. Forthcoming.
7. Davidson, J. M.; Chen, J.; Crapo, L.; Gray, G.; Greenleaf, W. J.; and Catania, J. A. 1983. Hormonal changes and sexual function in aging men. *J Clin Endocrinol Metab.* In press July issue.
8. Dennerstein, L.; Burrows, G.; Wood, C.; and Hyman, G. 1980. Hormones and sexuality: effect of estrogen and progestogen. *Obstet Gynecol* 56:316–22.
9. Easley, E. B. 1978. Sex problems after the menopause. *Clinics in Obstet & Gynecol* 21:269–77.
10. Erickson, B. E. 1979. Emotional, sexual and hormonal differences in women with long and short menses. In *The Eastern Conference on Reproductive Behavior.* New Orleans: Tulane University.
11. Fedor-Freybergh, P. 1977. The influence of oestrogens on the well being and mental performance in climacteric and postmenopausal women. *Acta Obstet et Gynecol Scand* suppl. 64:1–64.
12. Gonzalez, E. R. 1980. Vitamin E report. *JAMA* Sept. 5, 1077–78.
13. Gruis, M. L., and Wagner, N. N. 1979. Sexuality during the cimacteric. *Postgrad Medicine* 65:197–207.
14. Hallstrom, T. 1977. Sexuality in the climacteric. *Clinics in Obstet & Gynecol* 4: 227–39.
15. Harman, S. M., and Tsitouras, P. D. 1980. Reproductive hormones in aging men I: measurement of sex steroids, basal luteinizing hormone, and leydig cell response to human chorionic gonadotropin. *J Clin Endocrinol Metab* 51:35–40.
16. Henker, F. C. 1977. A male climacteric syndrome: sexual, psychic and physical complaints in 50 middle-aged men. *Psychosomatics* 18:23–27.
17. Hite, S. 1976. *The Hite report.* New York: Macmillan.
18. Kinsey, A.; Pomeroy, W.; and Martin, C. 1953. *Sexual behavior in the human female.* Philadelphia: Saunders.
19. Masters, W., and Johnson, V. 1970. *Human sexual inadequacy.* Boston: Little Brown.
20. ———. 1966. *Human sexual response.* Boston: Little Brown.

21. Neugarten, B. L.; Wood, V.; Kraines, R. J.; and Loomis, B. 1963. Women's attitudes toward the menopause. *Vita Humana* 6:140–51.
22. Notelovitz, M. 1978. Gynecologic problems of menopausal women: part 3. Changes in extragenital tissues and sexuality. *Geriatrics* 78:51–58.
23. Pfeiffer, E.; Verwoerdt, A.; and Davis, G. 1972. Sexual behavior in middle life. *Am J Psychiat* 128:1262–67.
24. Studd, J. W. W.; Collins, W. P.; Chakravarti, S.; Newton, J. R.; Oram, D.; and Parsons, A. 1977. Oestradiol and testosterone implants in the treatment of psychosexual problems in the postmenopausal woman. *Br J Obstet Gynaecol* 84:314–16.
25. Utian, W. H. S. 1972. The true clinical features of postmenopause and oophorectomy and their response to oestrogen therapy. *S Afr Med J* 46:732–37.

Chapter 8   Hysterectomy

1. Amias, A. G. 1975. Sexual life after gynaecological operations. *Br Med J* 2:608–9.
2. Andrews, M. C., and Wentz, A. C. 1975. The effects of danazol on gonadotropins and steroid blood levels in normal and anovulatory women. *Am J Obstet Gynecol* 121:817–28.
3. Annegers, J. F.; Strom, H.; Decker, D. G.; Dockerty, H. B.; and O'Fallon, W. 1979. Ovarian cancer: incidence and case-control study. *Cancer* 43:723–29.
4. Backstrom, T., and Boyle, H. 1980. Persistence of premenstrual tension symptoms in hysterectomized women. Forthcoming.
5. Ballinger, C. B. 1975. Psychiatric morbidity and the menopause: screening of general population sample. *Br Med J* 3:344–46.
6. Barker, M. C. 1968. Psychiatric illness after hysterectomy. *Br Med J* 2:91–95.
7. Bunker, J. P. 1976. Elective hysterectomy—pro and con: public-health rounds at the Harvard School of Public Health. *NEJM* 295:264–68.
8. Burch, J. C.; Byrd, B. F.; and Vaughn, W. K. 1975. The effects of long-term estrogen administration to women following hysterectomy. *Front Horm Res* 3:208–14.
9. Byrd, B. F., Jr.; Burch, J. C.; and Vaughn, W. K. 1977. The impact of long term estrogen support after hysterectomy: a report of 1016 cases. *Ann Surg* 185:574–80.
10. Callantine, M. R., and Martin, P. L. 1975. Micronized 17 beta estradiol for oral estrogen therapy in menopausal women. *Obstet Gynecol* 46:37–41.
11. Centerwall, B. S. 1981. Premenopausal hysterectomy and cardiovascular disease. *Am J Obstet Gynecol* 139:58–61.
12. Coppen, A.; Bisshop, M.; Beard, R. J. H.; Barnard, G. J. R.; and Collins, W. P. 1981. Hysterectomy, hormones, and behavior. *Lancet* 126–128.
13. Craig, G. A., and Jackson, P. 1975. Letter: sexual life after vaginal hysterectomy. *Br Med J* 3:97.
14. Cutler, W. B., and García, C.-R. 1983. Sexual deficits and hysterectomy: a reappraisal and review. In press.
15. Dalton, K. 1957. Discussion on the aftermath of hysterectomy and oophorectomy. *Proc Royal Soc of Med* 50:415–18.

16. DeNeef, J. C., and Hollenbeck, Z. J. R. 1966. The fate of ovaries preserved at the time of hysterectomy. *Am J Obstet Gynecol* 96:1088–97.
17. Dennerstein, L.; Wood, D.; and Burrows, G. 1977. Sexual response following hysterectomy and oophorectomy. *Obstet Gynecol* 49:92–96.
18. Dicker, R. C.; Scally, M. J.; Greenspan, J. R.; Layde, P. M.; and Maze, J. M. 1982. Hysterectomy among women of reproductive age. *JAMA* 248:323–27.
19. Donahue, V. C. 1976. Elective hysterectomy: pro and con. *NEJM* 295:264.
20. Doyle, L. I.; Barclay, D. L.; Duncan, G. W.; and Kirton, K. T. 1971. Human luteal function as assessed by plasma progestin. *Am J Obstet Gynecol* 110:92–97.
21. Forney, J. P. 1980. The effect of radical hysterectomy on bladder physiology. *Am J Obstet Gynecol* 138:374–82.
22. Gambrell, R. D.; Castaneda, T. A.; and Ricci, C. A. 1978. Management of postmenopausal bleeding to prevent endometrial cancer. *Maturitas* 1:99–106.
23. García C.-R., and Rosenfeld, D. L. 1977. *Human fertility: the regulation of reproduction.* Philadelphia: F. A. Davis.
24. Gath, D. H. 1980. Psychiatric aspects of hysterectomy. In *The social consequences of non-psychiatric illness.* New York: Bruner/Mazel.
25. Greenberg, M. 1981. Hysterectomy, hormones and behavior: letter to the editor. *Lancet* 449.
26. Hasselquist, M.; Goldberg, N.; Schroeter, A.; and Spelsberg, T. 1980. Isolation and characterization of the estrogen receptors in human skin. *J Clin Endocrinol Metab* 50:76–82.
27. Hempel, Von E.; Kriester, A.; Freesmeyer, E.; and Walter, W. 1979. Prospektive studie zur osteoporose nach bilater ovarektomie mit und ohne postoperative ostrogen-prophylaxe. *Zentralblatt für gynakologie* 101:309–19.
28. Hunter, D. J.; Julier, D.; Franklin, M.; and Green, E. 1977. Plasma levels of estrogen, luteinizing hormone, and follicle stimulating hormone following castration and estradiol implant. *Obstet Gynecol* 49:180–85.
29. Janson, P. O., and Jansson, I. 1977. The acute effect of hysterectomy on ovarian blood flow. *Am J Obstet Gynecol* 127:349–52.
30. Jick, H.; Dinan, B.; and Rotheman, K. 1978. Noncontraceptive estrogens and nonfatal myocardial infarctions. *JAMA* 239:1407–8 and subsequent personal communication.
31. Johnson, J. 1982. Tubal sterilization and hysterectomy. *Family Planning Perspectives* 14:28–30.
32. Knapp, R. C.; Donahue, V. C.; and Friedman, E. A. 1973. Dissection of paravesical and pararectal spaces in pelvic operations. *Surg Gynecol Obstet* 137:758–62.
33. Laros, R. K., and Work, B. A. 1975. Female sterilization III: vaginal hysterectomy. *Am J Obstet Gynecol* 122:693–97.
34. Lewis, E., and Bourne, S. 1981. Hysterectomy, hormones and behavior: letter to the editor. *Lancet* 324–25.
35. Longcope, C.; Hunter, R.; and Franz, C. 1980. Steroid secretion by the postmenopausal ovary. *Am J Obstet Gynecol* 138:564–68.

36. Lyon, L. J., and Gardner, J. W. 1977. The rising frequency of hysterectomy: its effect on uterine cancer rates. *Am J Epidemiol* 105:439–43.

37. MacManon, B., and Worcester, J. 1966. National center for health statistics: age at menopause, US 1960–1962. Washington, D.C., USPHS publication 1000, series 11, no. 19.

38. McNatty, K. P.; Makris, A.; DeGrazia, C.; Osathanondh, R.; and Ryan, K. J. 1979. The production of progesterone, androgens, and estrogens by granulosa cells, thecal tissue and stromal tissue by human ovaries in vitro. *J Clin Endocrinol Metab* 49: 687–99.

39. Mikhail, G. 1970. Hormone secretion by the human ovaries. *Gynec Invest* 1:5–20.

40. Monroe, S. E., and Menon, K. M. J. 1977. Changes in reproductive hormone secretion during the climacteric and postmenopausal periods. *Clinics in Obstet & Gynecol* 20:113–22.

41. Moore, J., and Tolley, D. 1976. Depression following hysterectomy. *Psychosomatics* 17:86–89.

42. Morgan, S. 1980. Sexuality after hysterectomy and castration. Published in offpress collection of women's writings.

43. Perry, J. D., and Whipple, B. 1981. Pelvic muscle strength of female ejaculators: evidence in support of a new theory of orgasm. *J Sex Res* 17:22–39.

44. Polivy, J. 1974. Psychological reactions to hysterectomy. *Am J Obstet Gynecol* 118: 417–26.

45. Punonen, R., and Rauramo, L. 1977. The effect of long-term oral oestriol succinate therapy on the skin of castrated women. *Ann Chir Gynaecol* 66:214–15.

46. Randall, C. L. 1963. Ovarian conservation. In *Progress in gynecology,* ed. J. V. Meigs and S. H. Sturgis, pp. 457–64. New York: Grune & Stratton.

47. Ranney, B., and Abu-Ghazaleh, S. 1977. The future function and control of ovarian tissue which is retained in vivo during hysterectomy. *Am J Obstet Gynecol* 128: 626–34.

48. Reynoso, R. L.; Aznar, R. R.; Bedolla, T. N.; and Cortes Gallego, V. 1975. Cyclic concentration of estradiol and progestone in hysterectomized women. *Reproduction* 2:45–49.

49. Richards, B. C. 1978. Hysterectomy: from women to women. *Am J Obstet Gynecol* 131:446–49.

50. Richards, D. H. 1973. Depression after hysterectomy. *Lancet* 2:430–33.

51. ———. 1974. A post hysterectomy syndrome. *Lancet* 983–85.

52. Ritterband, A. B.; Jaffe, I. A.; Densen, P. M.; Magagna, J. F.; and Reed, E. 1963. Gonadal function and the development of coronary heart disease. *Circulation* 27: 237–44.

53. Rivin, A. U., and Dimitroff, S. P. 1954. The incidence and severity of atherosclerosis in estrogen treated males and in females with a hypoestrogenic or hyperestrogenic state. *Circulation* 9:533–39.

54. Robinson, R. W.; Higano, N.; and Coehn, W. D. 1959. Increased incidence of coronary heart disease in women castrated prior to menopause. *Arch Intern Med* 104:908–11.

55. Rosenberg, L.; Hennekens, C. H.; Rosner, B.; Belanger, C.; Rothman, K. J.; and Speizer, R. E. 1981. Early menopause and the risk of myocardial infarction. *Am J Obstet Gynecol* 139:47–51.

56. Simon, J. A., and di Zerega, G. S. 1982. Physiologic estradiol replacement following oophorectomy: failure to maintain precastration gonadotropin levels. *Obstet Gynecol* 59:511–13.

57. Stadel, B. V., and Weiss, N. 1975. Characteristics of menopausal women: a survey of King and Pierce Counties in Washington, 1973–1974. *Am J Epidemiol* 102: 209–16.

58. Stone, S. C.; Dickey, R. P.; and Mickal, A. 1975. The acute effect of hysterectomy on ovarian function. *Am J Obstet Gynecol* 121:193–97.

59. Studd, J. W. W.; Chakravarti, S.; and Collins, W. P. 1978. Plasma hormone profiles after the menopause and bilateral oophorectomy. *Postgrad Med J* 54:25–30.

60. Tobachman, J. K.; Tucker, M. A.; Kase, R.; Greene, M. K.; Costa, J.; and Fraumeni, J. F., Jr. 1982. Intra abdominal carcinomatosis after prophylactic oophorectomy in ovarian cancer prone families. *Lancet* 795–97.

61. Treloar, A. 1981. Menstrual cyclicity and the pre menopause. *Maturitas* 3:249–64.

62. Utian, W. H. 1975. Definitive symptoms of postmenopause—incorporating use of vaginal parabasal cell index. *Front Horm Res* 3:74–93.

63. ———. 1975. Effect of hysterectomy, oophorectomy and estrogen therapy on libido. *Int J Obstet Gyn* 13:97–100.

64. Waldron, I. 1982. An analysis of causes of sex differences in mortality and morbidity. In *The fundamental connection between nature and nurture*, eds. W. R. Gove and G. R. Carpenter. Lexington, Mass.: Lexington Books.

65. ———. 1980. Employment and women's health: an analysis of causal relationships. *Int J Health Services* 10:435–54.

66. White, S. C.; Wartel, L. J.; and Wade, M. E. 1971. Comparison of abdominal and vaginal hysterectomies: a review of 600 operations. *Obstet Gynecol* 37:530–37.

67. Wright, R. C. 1969. Hysterectomy: past, present and future. *Obstet Gynecol* 33: 560–63.

68. Wuest, J. H.; Dry, T. J.; and Edwards, J. E. 1953. The degree of atherosclerosis in bilaterally oophorectomized women. *Circulation* 7:801–9.

69. Zussman, L.; Zussman, S.; Sunley, R.; and Bjornson, E. 1981. Sexual response after hysterectomy-oophorectomy: recent studies and reconsideration of psychogenesis. *Am J Obstet Gynecol* 140:725–29.

Appendix 1

1. Bye, P. B. 1978. Review of the status of oestrogen replacement therapy. *Postgrad Med J* 54:7–10.

2. Callantine, M. R.; Martin, P. L.; Bolding, O. T.; Warner, P. O.; and Greaney, M. O., Jr. 1975. Micronized 17 beta estradiol for oral estrogen therapy in menopausal women. *Obstet Gyencol* 46:37–41.

3. Campbell, S., and Whitehead, M. 1977. Oestrogen therapy and the menopausal syndrome. *Clinics in Obstet & Gynecol* 4:31–47.
4. Claydon, J. R.; Bell, J. Y.; and Pilard, P. 1974. Menopausal flushing: double blind trial of a non hormonal medication. *Br Med J* 1:409–12.
5. Dennerstein, L.; Burrow, G.; and Hyman, G. 1978. Menopausal hot flushes: a double blind comparison of placebo, ethinyl oestradiol and norgestrel. *Br J Obstet Gynaecol* 85:852–56.
6. Hunter, D. J.; Julier, D.; Franklin, M.; and Green, E. 1977. Plasma levels of estrogen, luteinizing hormone, and follicle stimulating hormone following castration and estradiol implant. *Obstet Gynecol* 49:180–85.
7. Kupperman, H. S.; Wetchler, B. B.; and Blatt, M. H. G. 1959. Contemporary therapy of the menopausal syndrome. *JAMA* 171:1627–37.
8. Larsson-Cohn, U.; Johansson, E. D.; Kagedal, B.; and Wallentin, L. 1977. Serum FSH, LH, and oestrone levels in postmenopausal patients on oestrogen therapy. *Br J Obstet Gynaecol* 85:367–72.
9. Lauritzen, C. 1973. The management of the premenopausal and the postmenopausal patient. *Front Horm Res* 2:2–21.
10. Lind, T.; Cameron, E. C.; Hunter, W. M.; Leon, C.; Moran, P. F.; Oxley, A.; Gerrard, J.; and Lind, U. C. G. 1979. A prospective controlled trial of six forms of hormone replacement therapy given to postmenopausal women. *Br J Obstet Gynaecol* 86, suppl. 3:1–29.
11. Lindsay, R., and Hart, D. M. 1978. Failure of response of menopausal vasomotor symptoms to clonidine. *Maturitas* 1:21–25.
12. Martin, P.; Yen, S. S. C.; Burnier, A. M.; and Hermann, H. 1979. Systemic absorption and sustained effects of vaginal estrogen creams. *JAMA* 242:2699–2700.
13. Tzingounis, V.; Aksu, M.; and Greenblatt, R. 1978. Estriol in the management of the menopause. *JAMA* 239:1638–41.

Appendix 2

1. Aylward, M. 1978. Coagulation factors in opposed and unopposed oestrogen treatment at the climacteric. *Postgrad Med J* 54:31–37.
2. Barret-Conner, E.; Brown, V.; Turner, J.; Austin, M. S.; and Criqui, M. H. 1979. Heart disease risk factors and hormone use in postmenopausal women. *JAMA* 20:2167–69.
3. Bolton, C. H.; Ellwood, M., Hartog, M.; Martin, R.; Rowe, A. S.; and Wensley, R. T. 1975. Comparison of the effects of ethinyl oestradiol and conjugated equine oestrogens in oophorectomized women. *Clin Endocrin (Oxf)* 4:131–38.
4. Bradley, D. B.; Wingerd, J.; and Petitti, D. B. 1978. Serum high density lipoprotein cholesterol in women using oral contraceptives, estrogens and progestins. *NEJM* 299:17–20.
5. Burch, J. C.; Byrd, B. F.; and Vaughn, W. K. 1975. The effects of long-term estrogen administration to women following hysterectomy. *Front Horm Res* 3:208–14.

228 BIBLIOGRAPHY

6. Campbell, S., and Whitehead, M. 1977. Oestrogen therapy and the menopausal syndrome. *Clinics in Obstet & Gynecol* 4:31–47.
7. Christiansen, C.; Christensen, M. S.; Hagen, C.; Stocklund, K. E.; and Transbol, I. 1981. Effects of natural estrogen/gestagen and thiazide on coronary risk factors in normal postmenopausal women. *Acta Obstet et Gynecol Scand* 60:407–12.
8. Crane, M. G.; Harris, J. J.; and Winsor, W. I. 1971. Hypertensions, oral contraceptive agents and conjugated estrogens. *Ann Int Med* 74:13–21.
9. Fedor-Freybergh, P. 1977. The influence of estrogens on the well-being and mental performance in the climacterica and postmenopausal women. *Acta Obstet et Gynecol Scand* 64, suppl. 1:1–64.
10. Gordon, T.; Kanel, W.; Hjortland, M.; and McNamara, P. 1978. Menopause and coronary heart disease: the Framingham Study. *Ann Int Med* 89:157–61.
11. Hirvonen, E.; Malknonen, M.; and Nanninen, V. 1980. Effects of different progestogens on lipoproteins during postmenopausal replacement therapy. *NEJM* 304:560–63.
12. Jick, H.; Dinan, B.; and Rothman, K. 1978. Noncontraceptive estrogens and nonfatal myocardial infarctions. *JAMA* 239:1407–8.
13. Kannel, W. B.; Castelli, W. P.; Gordon, T.; and McNamara, P. 1971. Serum cholesterol, lipoproteins and the risk of coronary heart disease. *Ann Int Med* 174:1 ff.
14. Lauritzen, C. 1973. The management of the premenopausal and the postmenopausal patient. *Front Horm Res* 2:2–21.
15. Lind, T.; Cameron, E. C.; Hunter, W. M.; Leon, C.; Moran, P. F.; Oxley, A.; Gerrard, J.; and Lind, U. C. G. 1979. A prospective controlled trial of six forms of hormone replacement therapy given to postmenopausal women. *Br J Obstet Gynaecol* 86, suppl. 3:1–29.
16. MacMahon, B. 1978. Oestrogen replacement therapy and the vascular risk. In *Coronary heart disease in young women*, pp. 197–207. Edinburgh: Churchill Livingstone.
17. Maddock, J. 1978. Effects of progestogens on serum lipids in the postmenopause. *Postgrad Med J* 54:367–70.
18. Miller, N. E. 1979. The evidence for the antiatherogenicity of high density lipoprotein in man. *Lipids* 13:914–19.
19. Nielson, F. H.; Honore, E.; Kristoffersen, K.; Secher, N. J.; and Pederson, G. T. 1977. Changes in serum lipids during treatment with norgestrel, oestradiol-valerate and cyclprogynon. *Acta Obstet et Gynecol Scand* 56:367–370.
20. Notelovitz, M. 1977. Coagulation, oestrogen and the menopause. *Clinics in Obstet & Gynecol* 4:107–28.
21. Notelovitz, M., and Southwood, B. 1974. Metabolic effect of conjugated equine oestrogens (USP) on lipids and lipoproteins. *S Afr Med J* 48:2552–56.
22. Pfeffer, R. I., and van den Noort, S. S. 1976. Estrogen use and stroke risk in postmenopausal women. *Am J Epidemiol* 103:445–56.
23. Pfeffer, R. I.; Whipple, G. H.; Kurosaki, T. T.; and Chapman, J. M. 1978. Coronary risk and estrogen use in postmenopausal women. *Am J Epidemiol* 107:479–87.
24. Plunkett, E. R. 1982. Contraceptive steroids, age and the cardiovascular system. *Am J Obstet Gynecol* 142:747–51.

25. Punnonen, R., and Rauramo, L. 1976. The effect of castration and oral estrogen therapy on serum lipids. In *Concensus on menopause research*, ed. P. A. van Keep and R. B. Greenblatt, pp. 132–38. Baltimore: University Park Press.

26. Pyorala, T. 1976. The effect of synthetic and natural estrogens on glucose tolerance, plasma insulin and lipid metabolism in postmenopausal women. In *The management of the menopause and postmenopausal years*, ed. S. Campbell, pp. 195–210. Lancaster, Eng.: MTP Press.

27. Rosenberg, L.; Armstrong, B.; and Jick, H. 1976. Myocardial infarction and estrogen therapy in postmenopausal women. *NEJM* 294:1256–59.

28. Ross, R. K.; Paganini-Hill, A.; Mack, T. M.; Arthur, M.; and Henderson, B. 1981. Menopausal estrogen therapy and protection from death from ischaemic heart disease. *Lancet* 1:858–60.

29. Saunders, D. M.; Hunter, J. C.; Shutt, D. A.; and O'Neill, B. J. 1978. The effect of oestradiol valerate therapy on coagulation factors and lipid and oestrogen levels in oophorectomized women. *Aust N Z J Obstet Gynaecol* 18:198–201.

30. Silverstolpe, G.; Gustafson, A.; Samsioe, G.; and Svanborg, A. 1979. Lipid metabolic studies in oophorectomized women: effects of three different progestogens. *Acta Obstet et Gynecol Scand* suppl., 88:89–95.

31. Tikkanen, M. J.; Juusi, T.; et al. 1979. Treatment of post-menopausal hypercholesterolaemia with estradiol. *Acta Obstet et Gynecol Scand* suppl., 88:83–88.

32. Tikkanen, M. J., and Nikkila, E. A. 1978. Natural oestrogen as an effective treatment for type-11 hyperlipoproteinaemia in postmenopausal women. *Lancet* 490–501.

33. Toy, J. L.; Davies, J. A.; and McNicol, G. P. 1978. The effects of long term therapy with oestriol succinate on the haemostatic mechanism in postmenopausal women. *Br J Obstet Gynaecol* 85:363–66.

34. Utian, W. H. 1978. Effect of postmenopausal estrogen therapy on diastolic blood pressure and bodyweight. *Maturitas* 1:3–8.

35. Wallace, R. B.; Hoover, J.; Barrett-Connor, E.; Rifkind, B. M.; Hunninghake, D. B.; Mackenthun, A.; and Heiss, G. 1979. Altered plasma lipid and lipoprotein levels associated with oral contraceptive and oestrogen use. *Lancet* July 21, 111–15.

36. Wallentin, L., and Larsson-Cohn, U. 1977. Metabolic and hormonal effects of postmenopausal oestrogen replacement treatment, II: plasma lipid. *Acta Endocrinol* 86: 597–607.

37. Walter, S., and Jensen, H. K. 1977. The effect of treatment with oestradiol and oestriol on fasting serum cholesterol and triglyceride levels in postmenopausal women. *Br J Obstet Gynaecol* 84:869–72.

Glossary

androgen: a class of male sex hormones that both men and women have, although men have more.

androstenedione: a weak androgen that menopausal ovaries secrete abundantly, as do the adrenals. This hormone becomes a major source of menopausal estrogens because it is changed into estrogens by the fat cells of the body.

atherosclerosis: hardening of the arteries.

atrophic: deteriorating cells.

bilateral salpingo ovariectomy: surgical removal of both ovaries and oviducts.

cervix: the neck of the uterus, which sits on the internal end of the vagina.

coitus: sexual connection per vagina between male and female.

corpus luteum: the "yellow body" seen in the ovary after ovulation. Its cells produce progesterone and estrogen (in the human) as well as other hormones.

D & C: dilatation and curettage. The process by which a physician opens (dilates) the entry to the uterus and then scrapes away the lining (endometrium) of the uterus.

detumescence: loss of swelling as in loss of penile erection.

double-blind study: a study in which neither the experimenter nor the subject knows who is getting what treatment until all the results are in.

dyspareunia: difficult or painful coitus. A common condition when the vagina is not able to form lubrication adequately. Common when menopausal estrogen deficiency progresses.

endocrine gland: *see* gland (endocrine).

endometrium: the lining portion of the uterus. A complex tissue that changes in size and composition throughout the menstrual cycle each month, forming a thick and cushiony mass of cells in preparation for a potential fertilized egg. Should none arrive, the endometrium itself sloughs off and is washed away with the menstrual flow. With estrogen deficiencies, the endometrium becomes thin and atrophic.

ERT: estrogen replacement therapy.

estradiol: the strongest of the estrogens.

estriol: the weakest commonly found estrogen.

estrogen: a class of female sex hormones that both men and women have, although women have more.

estrone: a weaker estrogen than estradiol.

Fallopian tubes: the two tubes that connect the ovaries with the uterus, and through which sperm enters to fertilize an egg and an egg travels to reach the uterus.

gland (endocrine): a part of the body (for example, adrenals, ovaries) that manufactures hormones and releases them into the blood stream.

hemorrhage: abnormal internal or external bleeding.

high-density lipoprotein: formed of protein coupled to a fat droplet, this molecule, which travels in the blood stream, protects against heart disease.

hormone: a substance produced in a gland that can travel in the blood stream and exert action on cells in a different part of the body than where it was produced.

hormone replacement therapy: *see* HRT.

hot flush or flash: a sudden and quickly passing sensation of intense internal heat, followed by sweating and possibly a brief chill. Common at the menopause.

HRT: hormone replacement therapy (generally includes progesterone that is given with estrogen).

hypertension: high blood pressure usually more than 140/90.

hypertrophy: excessive swelling or increased size of tissue.

hysterectomy: removal of the uterus (not the ovary).

incontinent: unable to control urine retention.

LH: *see* luteinizing hormone.

libido: sexual appetite.

lipid: fatty substances that can't dissolve in blood.

lipoprotein: a substance traveling in the blood stream that is part lipid and part protein.

low-density lipoprotein: a lipoprotein with less protein and more lipid, as compared to the high density lipoprotein. High concentrations of this substance appear to promote heart disease.

luteinizing hormone: a hormone produced in the pituitary. A large surge of this hormone precedes ovulation by twelve to twenty-four hours each cycle.

menarche: the first menstrual period of a girl's life.

menopause: the time that follows the last menstrual period of a woman's life.

natural hormones: hormones that are chemically identical to those that occur in nature. (In contrast, see synthetic hormones.)

nulliparous: never having borne a child.

oophorectomy: removal of the ovary. Also called ovariectomy.

osteoporosis: increased porosity of bones. A disease found in estrogen deficiency states, which leads to bone fractures.

ovariectomy: *see* oophorectomy.

ovary: one of two female organs that contain the eggs and the cells which produce the female hormones estrogen and progesterone.

perimenopause: the time "around" the menopause during which menstrual cycles become irregular and often menopausal distress symptoms appear.

placebo: a pill that has no active ingredients.

progesterone: a hormone produced in the ovary principally by the corpus luteum

progestin: a hormone that has progesterone-like effects.

progestin challenge test: a way to check if progestins are needed.

prospective study: a study in which records are kept as a treatment continues. This is done to insure accuracy.

retrospective study: a study in which subjects remember what happened because records were not kept.

subtotal hysterectomy: removal of the uterus except for the cervix portion.

synthetic hormones: hormones that are chemically different from those that occur in nature.

testosterone: the strongest of the male sex hormones. Women also produce testosterone, though much less than men.

titration: the addition of small increments until the correct balance is achieved.

total abdominal hysterectomy: removal of the total uterus by abdominal surgery. Does not include oophorectomy.

total hysterectomy: removal of the total uterus.

unopposed estrogen: estrogen treatment without progestin opposition, which is usually recommended.

uterus: a complex female organ composed of smooth muscle and glandular lining.

vagina: a muscular canal in the female that extends from the vulva to the cervix. It is very responsive to estrogen and becomes atrophied during menopausal estrogen deficiency states.

vaginitis: inflammation of the vagina. It is marked by pain, discharge, and itchiness.

womb: the uterus.

Index

235

Annual Health Charts

The pages that follow are designed as a personal diary for recording the facts about your passage through and beyond the change of life. By recording your days of menstruation, symptoms, treatments, and other medical history, you will provide useful diagnostic tools.

If you are methodical and orderly in keeping an accurate record of your health habits and needs, you will begin a journey into awareness that will help detect problems earlier and will aid you in achieving a happier, healthier, and more productive life. The seven years before your last period are generally characterized by a number of changes in menstrual pattern. It helps to record days of bleeding in order to see the change over time. Beginning at about age forty-three, changes generally become apparent. Figure 20 presents a sample Menstrual Record Form. If you decide to use it, it will help future diagnosis if you note the character of the blood flow. If other forms than those designated in the code occur

Name:

Age:

Current Year:

MENSTRUAL RECORD CHART

Month	1	2	3	4	5	6	7	8	9	10	11	12	13	14	15	16	17	18	19	20	21	22	23	24	25	26	27	28	29	30	31
JAN																															
FEB																															
MARCH																															
APRIL																															
MAY																															
JUNE																															
JULY																															
AUG																															
SEPT																															
OCT																															
NOV																															
DEC																															

Don't forget to have this chart with you when you call or visit your doctor.

TYPE OF FLOW: Normal ☒   Light ◙   Heavy ■   Stain ◙

Figure 20 Menstrual History

(for example, clots), make up your own code letter and add that code letter whenever they occur.

Space is provided in the following pages to allow a permanent record, one page for each year—starting now. This record will help you as well as your daughters and granddaughters. It is easy to jot things down as they happen but difficult to remember them accurately after time has passed.

Name:

Age:

Current Year:

MENSTRUAL RECORD CHART

Month	1	2	3	4	5	6	7	8	9	10	11	12	13	14	15	16	17	18	19	20	21	22	23	24	25	26	27	28	29	30	31
JAN																															
FEB																															
MARCH																															
APRIL																															
MAY																															
JUNE																															
JULY																															
AUG																															
SEPT																															
OCT																															
NOV																															
DEC																															

Don't forget to have this chart with you when you call or visit your doctor.

TYPE OF FLOW: Normal ☒   Light ▣   Heavy ■   Stain ▣

ANNUAL HEALTH CHART   FOR THE YEAR _____

	Jan.	Feb.	March	April	May	June	July	Aug.	Sept.	Oct.	Nov.	Dec.
Illnesses:												
Surgeries:												
Injuries:												
Medications and immunizations:												
Symptoms:												

Name:

Age:

Current Year:

MENSTRUAL RECORD CHART

Month	1	2	3	4	5	6	7	8	9	10	11	12	13	14	15	16	17	18	19	20	21	22	23	24	25	26	27	28	29	30	31
JAN																															
FEB																															
MARCH																															
APRIL																															
MAY																															
JUNE																															
JULY																															
AUG																															
SEPT																															
OCT																															
NOV																															
DEC																															

Don't forget to have this chart with you when you call or visit your doctor.

TYPE OF FLOW: Normal ⊠ Light ▣ Heavy ■ Stain ▣

FOR THE YEAR _____

	Jan.	Feb.	March	April	May	June	July	Aug.	Sept.	Oct.	Nov.	Dec.
Illnesses:												
Surgeries:												
Injuries:												
Medications and immunizations:												
Symptoms:												

Name:

Age:

Current Year:

MENSTRUAL RECORD CHART

Month	1	2	3	4	5	6	7	8	9	10	11	12	13	14	15	16	17	18	19	20	21	22	23	24	25	26	27	28	29	30	31
JAN																															
FEB																															
MARCH																															
APRIL																															
MAY																															
JUNE																															
JULY																															
AUG																															
SEPT																															
OCT																															
NOV																															
DEC																															

Don't forget to have this chart with you when you call or visit your doctor.

TYPE OF FLOW: Normal ⊠   Light ◙   Heavy ■   Stain ◙

ANNUAL HEALTH CHART   FOR THE YEAR _____

	Jan.	Feb.	March	April	May	June	July	Aug.	Sept.	Oct.	Nov.	Dec.
Illnesses:												
Surgeries:												
Injuries:												
Medications and immunizations:												
Symptoms:												

Name:

Age:

Current Year:

MENSTRUAL RECORD CHART

Month	1	2	3	4	5	6	7	8	9	10	11	12	13	14	15	16	17	18	19	20	21	22	23	24	25	26	27	28	29	30	31
JAN																															
FEB																															
MARCH																															
APRIL																															
MAY																															
JUNE																															
JULY																															
AUG																															
SEPT																															
OCT																															
NOV																															
DEC																															

Don't forget to have this chart with you when you call or visit your doctor.

TYPE OF FLOW: Normal ☒   Light ▣   Heavy ■   Stain ◉

ANNUAL HEALTH CHART   FOR THE YEAR ____

	Jan.	Feb.	March	April	May	June	July	Aug.	Sept.	Oct.	Nov.	Dec.
Illnesses:												
Surgeries:												
Injuries:												
Medications and immunizations:												
Symptoms:												

Name: Age: Current Year:

MENSTRUAL RECORD CHART

Month	1	2	3	4	5	6	7	8	9	10	11	12	13	14	15	16	17	18	19	20	21	22	23	24	25	26	27	28	29	30	31
JAN																															
FEB																															
MARCH																															
APRIL																															
MAY																															
JUNE																															
JULY																															
AUG																															
SEPT																															
OCT																															
NOV																															
DEC																															

Don't forget to have this chart with you when you call or visit your doctor.

TYPE OF FLOW: Normal ☒   Light ⊡   Heavy ■   Stain ⊡

	Jan.	Feb.	March	April	May	June	July	Aug.	Sept.	Oct.	Nov.	Dec.
Illnesses:												
Surgeries:												
Injuries:												
Medications and immunizations:												
Symptoms:												

Name:

Age: Current Year:

MENSTRUAL RECORD CHART

Month	1	2	3	4	5	6	7	8	9	10	11	12	13	14	15	16	17	18	19	20	21	22	23	24	25	26	27	28	29	30	31
JAN																															
FEB																															
MARCH																															
APRIL																															
MAY																															
JUNE																															
JULY																															
AUG																															
SEPT																															
OCT																															
NOV																															
DEC																															

Don't forget to have this chart with you when you call or visit your doctor.

TYPE OF FLOW: Normal ⊠   Light ◙   Heavy ■   Stain ◙

ANNUAL HEALTH CHART   FOR THE YEAR ___

	Jan.	Feb.	March	April	May	June	July	Aug.	Sept.	Oct.	Nov.	Dec.
Illnesses:												
Surgeries:												
Injuries:												
Medications and immunizations:												
Symptoms:												

Name: Current Year:

Age:

MENSTRUAL RECORD CHART

Month	1	2	3	4	5	6	7	8	9	10	11	12	13	14	15	16	17	18	19	20	21	22	23	24	25	26	27	28	29	30	31
JAN																															
FEB																															
MARCH																															
APRIL																															
MAY																															
JUNE																															
JULY																															
AUG																															
SEPT																															
OCT																															
NOV																															
DEC																															

Don't forget to have this chart with you when you call or visit your doctor.

TYPE OF FLOW: Normal ☒   Light ◙   Heavy ■   Stain ◙

	Jan.	Feb.	March	April	May	June	July	Aug.	Sept.	Oct.	Nov.	Dec.
Illnesses:												
Surgeries:												
Injuries:												
Medications and immunizations:												
Symptoms:												

Name:

Age: Current Year:

MENSTRUAL RECORD CHART

Month	1	2	3	4	5	6	7	8	9	10	11	12	13	14	15	16	17	18	19	20	21	22	23	24	25	26	27	28	29	30	31
JAN																															
FEB																															
MARCH																															
APRIL																															
MAY																															
JUNE																															
JULY																															
AUG																															
SEPT																															
OCT																															
NOV																															
DEC																															

Don't forget to have this chart with you when you call or visit your doctor.

TYPE OF FLOW: Normal ⊠   Light ⊡   Heavy ■   Stain ⊙

	Jan.	Feb.	March	April	May	June	July	Aug.	Sept.	Oct.	Nov.	Dec.
Illnesses:												
Surgeries:												
Injuries:												
Medications and immunizations:												
Symptoms:												

Name:

Age:

Current Year:

MENSTRUAL RECORD CHART

Month	1	2	3	4	5	6	7	8	9	10	11	12	13	14	15	16	17	18	19	20	21	22	23	24	25	26	27	28	29	30	31
JAN																															
FEB																															
MARCH																															
APRIL																															
MAY																															
JUNE																															
JULY																															
AUG																															
SEPT																															
OCT																															
NOV																															
DEC																															

Don't forget to have this chart with you when you call or visit your doctor.

TYPE OF FLOW: Normal ☒   Light ⊡   Heavy ■   Stain ⊡

FOR THE YEAR _____

	Jan.	Feb.	March	April	May	June	July	Aug.	Sept.	Oct.	Nov.	Dec.
Illnesses:												
Surgeries:												
Injuries:												
Medications and immunizations:												
Symptoms:												

Name:

Age:

Current Year:

MENSTRUAL RECORD CHART

Month	1	2	3	4	5	6	7	8	9	10	11	12	13	14	15	16	17	18	19	20	21	22	23	24	25	26	27	28	29	30	31
JAN																															
FEB																															
MARCH																															
APRIL																															
MAY																															
JUNE																															
JULY																															
AUG																															
SEPT																															
OCT																															
NOV																															
DEC																															

Don't forget to have this chart with you when you call or visit your doctor.

TYPE OF FLOW: Normal ⊠ Light ▣ Heavy ■ Stain ⊡

ANNUAL HEALTH CHART   FOR THE YEAR _____

	Jan.	Feb.	March	April	May	June	July	Aug.	Sept.	Oct.	Nov.	Dec.
Illnesses:												
Surgeries:												
Injuries:												
Medications and immunizations:												
Symptoms:												

Name:

Age:

Current Year:

MENSTRUAL RECORD CHART

Month	1	2	3	4	5	6	7	8	9	10	11	12	13	14	15	16	17	18	19	20	21	22	23	24	25	26	27	28	29	30	31
JAN																															
FEB																															
MARCH																															
APRIL																															
MAY																															
JUNE																															
JULY																															
AUG																															
SEPT																															
OCT																															
NOV																															
DEC																															

Don't forget to have this chart with you when you call or visit your doctor.

TYPE OF FLOW: Normal ☒   Light ◙   Heavy ■   Stain ◙

	Jan.	Feb.	March	April	May	June	July	Aug.	Sept.	Oct.	Nov.	Dec.
Illnesses:												
Surgeries:												
Injuries:												
Medications and immunizations:												
Symptoms:												

Name:

Age:

Current Year:

MENSTRUAL RECORD CHART

Month	1	2	3	4	5	6	7	8	9	10	11	12	13	14	15	16	17	18	19	20	21	22	23	24	25	26	27	28	29	30	31
JAN																															
FEB																															
MARCH																															
APRIL																															
MAY																															
JUNE																															
JULY																															
AUG																															
SEPT																															
OCT																															
NOV																															
DEC																															

Don't forget to have this chart with you when you call or visit your doctor.

TYPE OF FLOW: Normal ⊠   Light ⊡   Heavy ■   Stain ⊡

ANNUAL HEALTH CHART FOR THE YEAR _____

	Jan.	Feb.	March	April	May	June	July	Aug.	Sept.	Oct.	Nov.	Dec.
Illnesses:												
Surgeries:												
Injuries:												
Medications and immunizations:												
Symptoms:												

Name:

Age:

Current Year:

MENSTRUAL RECORD CHART

Month	1	2	3	4	5	6	7	8	9	10	11	12	13	14	15	16	17	18	19	20	21	22	23	24	25	26	27	28	29	30	31
JAN																															
FEB																															
MARCH																															
APRIL																															
MAY																															
JUNE																															
JULY																															
AUG																															
SEPT																															
OCT																															
NOV																															
DEC																															

Don't forget to have this chart with you when you call or visit your doctor.

TYPE OF FLOW: Normal ⊠   Light ▣   Heavy ■   Stain ◙

ANNUAL HEALTH CHART   FOR THE YEAR ____

	Jan.	Feb.	March	April	May	June	July	Aug.	Sept.	Oct.	Nov.	Dec.
Illnesses:												
Surgeries:												
Injuries:												
Medications and immunizations:												
Symptoms:												